Kin

"I am absolutely stun*
read from other sources, *many* ___
instinctively that every word is true. Other things I think I secretly already
knew, but could not bring myself to admit before. My eyes (and mind) became
clearer with each chapter. Like a fog lifting."
Paul White, London, UK

~~~

"If what is spoken about in *Fresh Wisdom* is true, then its brave founders,
have, knowingly put themselves at considerable risk to a world that is going
down a path of no return. For no Government likes to hear the truth."
Peter Fischer, Sydney, Australia

~~~

I have learned a lot from different (web) sites all over the world. I only wish I
had found *Fresh Wisdom* a year ago. With the wisdom I have acquired,
through study, I couldn't put it all together until now. I can't wait to see what
my life will be like now that I've read *Fresh Wisdom*.
Charles G. Dadley Jr., Lowell, MA, USA

~~~

I feel that I am now being equipped to cope with the world's misinformation
machine (mass-media) and misguided value system, among other 'mis'-
concepts we are bombarded with every day.
Geoff Hodskiss, Gold Coast, Queensland, Australia

~~~

There is a parallel universe that exists 180 degrees to the one in which our
minds currently reside, and it can be accessed in 10 seconds. The necessary
change is psychological. However, to perform this miracle, it is necessary to
understand the forces that bind us in this present realm of existence.
As near as I can discern, the authors of *Fresh Wisdom* have effectively learned
how to step outside this anti-civilization bubble where everyone is being
pushed from side to side, never knowing what is going on, or who is pulling
the strings, and view it from outside the bubble looking in.
Be prepared to have you paradigm challenged, but stick with it. Don't
overanalyze, and don't be concerned about things you don't understand
immediately. Stick with it to the conclusion and the pieces of the puzzle
should snap into place.
Ron Robinson, Salt Lake City, Utah, USA.
http://americanfreeenterprise.blogspot.com/2005/09/freedom-technology-
seminar-to-find-out.html

~~~

This seminar provides a 'sound bite' approach on some fundamental deceptions
and delusions. For the uninitiated, it hits hard (probably the only way to get
attention) and should provide much food for thought. Many thanks for making
this material available!
Serena Martin, London, UK

~~~

More Kind Words About Fresh Wisdom

I'm at the cross-roads of my life and I can tell you without mincing words that, your book is a REAL MIND-BLOWER. Accept my heartiest thanks and appreciation. Carry on the Good Work.
Nana Attobrah, France
~~~

I am a calculated and empathetic elitist entrepreneur. My sense of justice and truth has led me to you. Praises to you.
"Twisted Mirror", Dunedin, New Zealand
~~~

I've been surprised by the quality of your seminars and the clarity of thoughts regarding the current state of the world. The conclusions you have reached are similar to mine.
Lucian Ilea
~~~

In this day of fabricated evidence what more need one than the truth? I thank you for your hard work to help keep us free.
Michael Kahdushan
~~~

Finally, someone is willing to tell things as they are! Thank you Tony, Markus and Vicki for exposing in such a clear and logical manner the cons we've been subjected to and which unwittingly enslave us. It's long been my belief that the generally accepted definitions of success and a happy life leave much to be desired. You have at last explained why that is, and what it really means to lead a truly fulfilling life.
Fresh Wisdom is a breath of fresh air in a polluted world, where information abounds and REALITY is scarce. These are powerful, life-changing principles, if applied. And best of all they are easy to follow and make perfect sense, unlike other teachings I've come across in my travels.
I unhesitatingly recommend *Fresh Wisdom*. It is information like yours which has the potential to change the world. Unfortunately, though, few will recognize it as such and will pass on an opportunity to radically improve the quality of their life. You have a tough task ahead of you because of the already deeply ingrained propaganda we've been forcefully exposed to over 4 or more generations.
Michael Haupt, World Traveler, Contrarian Thinker and www.ThreeWorldWars.com Webmaster.
~~~

Fresh Wisdom is like taking both the blue pill and the red pill at the same time. You are still free to believe what you like (that is, accepted as you are) whilst the authors show you the consolidated realities in the world by having an open mind and how you can change or improve on them. *Fresh Wisdom* has both inspired and shown me how to walk the steps to freedom and what I need to be aware of during this process.
Peter Fischer, Sydney, Australia
~~~

Fresh Wisdom

Breakthrough to Enlightenment

Making Sense of Life in a Senseless World

Dr. Tony Hope
Markus Hart
Vicki Wilson

We want to hear from you. Please send your questions and comments about this book to fw@FreedomTechnology.org.

Freedom Technology Publishing

This title is also available as an audio recording. Visit www.freedomtechnology.org/audio for details.

First Published December 2005

ISBN 1-4196-1855-5

Printed and bound globally using the Print on Demand services of Book Surge Publishing LLC, a Division of Amazon.com

Visit Us Online at http://fw.FreedomTechnology.org
Contact Us by Email at fw@FreedomTechnology.org

To order additional copies, please contact us.
www.FreshWisdom.com
1-866-308-6235

This book is dedicated to you,
the Greatest Miracle of All.

It is no accident that you are
holding this book. This
magical moment was planned
long before you were born.
And the outcome of this
journey, too, is planned.

So sit back and enjoy the ride.

Obligatory Disclaimer:

This manual is provided with the understanding that the publisher, authors and advisors are not rendering legal, accounting, medical, marriage or any other professional advice or services.

You are encouraged to do your complete due diligence and research before applying any of the principles covered in this educational material. External references are supplied to aid this research.

Every effort has been made to make this manual as complete and accurate as possible and to ensure that the information was correct at the time of going to press. However, the authors and publisher do not assume and hereby disclaim any liability to any party for any loss or damage caused by errors or omissions, whether such errors or omissions result from negligence, accident or any other cause.

This manual should be used as a general guide, and not as the ultimate source of life instruction. Furthermore, this manual only contains information available prior to the publication date, and will not include information on any subsequent developments.

"Our deepest fear is not that we are inadequate. Our deepest fear is that we are powerful beyond measure. It is our light, not our darkness, that most frightens us.

We ask ourselves, "Who am I to be brilliant, gorgeous, talented and fabulous?"

Actually, who are you not to be? You are a child of God. Your playing small does not serve the world. There is nothing enlightened about shrinking so that other people will not feel insecure around you. We were born to manifest the glory of God that is within us. And as we let our own light shine, we unconsciously give other people permission to do the same.

As we are liberated from our own fear, our presence automatically liberates others." - Marianne Williamson (often incorrectly attributed to Nelson Mandela).

Table of Contents

1. Acknowledgements

The authors would like to acknowledge the hundreds of writers, teachers, philosophers and alternative thinkers, both classical and contemporary, who have unknowingly shaped our separate lives and brought us together after many years of searching. Their efforts have assisted in crystallizing these truths, and we thank God and you for the privilege of sharing them with you.

Special Mentions

- Ralph Epperson whose book *The Unseen Hand, An Introduction to the Conspiratorial View of History* assisted in understanding the Negative Force;
- Stuart Goldsmith whose *Inner Circle* material triggered the idea for the original Freedom Technology Email Seminar, from which this book is extracted;
- Frederick Mann of BuildFreedom.com – the modern day grandfather of freedom thinking;
- Helen and Aubrey Andelin, who woke us up to the reality of love, romance and correct gender roles in the 21st Century;
- John Eldredge for his mind-blowing explanation of 'spiritual sex' in *The Journey of Desire*;
- Harold and Arlene Brecher for providing ideas for renewed vitality;
- Steven Covey who best explained what it means to achieve a paradigm shift;
- John Reese who proved it really is possible to make $1million in 24 hours;
- Jay Abraham who taught us how to market the impossible;
- Our numerous advisors and counselors who watched this project from inception to launch and who provided much needed support, encouragement and reality checks;
- And the many other authors quoted in this manual.

We believe we have credited all works as required. If however you find an article or quote which has not been credited appropriately, please contact us so that the unintentional omission can be corrected immediately.

2. Getting the Most from This Manual

Do not for a minute think that this is a self-help book – this is a Life Manual which has great potential power beyond your wildest dreams. It will change your world view and can, as a result, forever alter your entire life. And we do not say that lightly.

By the end of this journey you will understand the bigger picture of life in this Universe, because we answer these and other similarly profound questions, using scientific proof and the Immutable Laws of Nature:

- Why are we here?
- What lies beyond the grave?
- How can we prepare for eternity?
- Where do we find an alternate reality?
- What is the Omega Point and how do we reach it?

Here are a few suggestions for getting the most out of this life-changing information.

First: Keep an open, rational, active mind. There are going to be a number of things which you will find shocking, disturbing or offensive in this book. This is quite intentional. Instead of dismissing something because it does not fit within your system, make a written entry of any questions, strong disagreements, severe discomfort, and examples which you think violate your system. But do not worry about these disagreements until you have completed the entire book. Many initial differences will have been answered as the complete picture unfolds.

Also keep in mind that we are not asking you to believe everything we say right away. Many think they must either accept or reject a new idea. There is a third alternative: reserve judgment. Think about things with an open, questioning mind as you continue reading - you will often find that what we say does have the ring of truth, because it conforms to the Immutable Laws of Nature.

Second: Start a journal. By reading this book, your life is about to change in ways you just cannot imagine right now. Many have told us how much they regret not keeping a record of changes in their lives. You may already know some of the information we are about to share, but there will be plenty of groundbreaking concepts discussed. You should record any new information to review in future. Since our brain retains information for longer when we write something down, we recommend a hand-written journal, but many have chosen to type their record instead.

There should be two parts to your journal: **Action Items** and **Points of Interest**. Action Items are any actions you can take immediately. Points of Interest are any new pieces of information which do not necessarily require action, but which you can keep in the back of your mind for future reference. Your Journal will be the most rewarding part of this manual – at the end of your journey you will be grateful for having kept one.

Third: Question and cross-check everything. We provide numerous external references and Internet links throughout this manual to back up many of the outrageous claims we make. Please take the time to validate what we say – this is *Fresh Wisdom's* 'self-checking mechanism'. Many find it easier to access the links from our website, as it is easier to click on an active link than type it into our browser. See www.FreedomTechnology.org/links.

We also refer to many other Freedom Technology resources. There is always a balance between Time and Money: more of one is less of the other. And so, while this manual will show you the principles of Fulfilled Living and how to do something for free, we will also show you where to get further help and guidance at a price that will be worth the time you can save. If you do not need further explanation or do not wish to save time, the recommendations can simply be ignored.

The manual is structured in such a way that we progress through various levels. A small percentage of readers are not surprised by anything we cover in early chapters and consider it rather obvious. This is because we must lay the groundwork and foundations first, in order to cater to widely differing levels of understanding.

Please bear with us as we bring other readers up to your level of understanding. By the time we have completed the basics of each of the 5 Essential Pillars of Fulfilled Living, we will be able to move ahead into the really challenging and exciting material.

We have the unique benefit of knowing from first hand experience (both our own and from feedback from others) that the journey you are about to commence is exciting, entertaining, unique and life changing.

It is a search for truth, in a world where truth no longer seems to exist.

Bear in mind Kahlil Gibran's words of wisdom in *The Prophet*:

> *"Say not, 'I have found the truth,' but rather, 'I have found a truth'"*.

Dr Auke J. Schade says:

> *"Absolute truth might be a temporary illusion. As scientific history shows, there are always new facts. Hence, the most recent facts are unlikely to be the absolute truth."[1]*

Come with us on a treasure hunt of time-tested Universal Principles. Once you understand the Principles, you do not need to study any details. You will know the details by knowing their principles. By the end of your roller-coaster ride you will have a collection of proven truths which you will use to reach your personal Omega Point.

As Lao Tzu says:

> *"Those who know are not learned;*
> *Those who are learned do not know."*

We hope you enjoy this journey of discovery. It has taken us thirty years of constant questioning to reach our Omega Point, and it is our sincere desire that you reach yours with far less effort and in a significantly quicker time. Here is your roadmap and travel guide to your personal Omega Point of perfect understanding.

We would love to hear about your travels. Send your adventures to fw@freedomtechnology.org.

---

[1] http://web.archive.org/web/20030213111734/www.dmmglobal.com/

3. Introduction

Fresh Wisdom is a hard-hitting exposé designed to identify the restrictive beliefs we have all unwittingly been forced to accept as truth, and which limit the freedom we could be enjoying. Understanding how much our thinking has been influenced by external parties allows us to take the next logical step of breaking free from those beliefs to a more fulfilled life. This journey is something very special, and at its conclusion you will be part of a unique group of *Fresh Thinkers*.

Trust

Together, we will build a bridge of trust between us. Because we provide proof along the way, you will come to trust us, and to believe that the information we share has 'the ring of truth', even though some of it may be difficult to accept at first.

We will come to trust you not to reveal these teachings to just anyone. There are dark and sinister forces, who for hundreds of years have purposely suppressed the truth, for their own misguided intentions. If word of *Fresh Wisdom* were to make its way into the wrong hands, this book could easily be banned and a lifetime of work will have been for nothing. Please be very careful who you share this information with, as we were in choosing a trusted, independent publisher.

All readers of *Fresh Wisdom* share one thing in common. They all desire to step out of the anti-civilization bubble encapsulating us and holding us back from being the person our Creator intended us to be. It came as no surprise to us that not everyone wants to attain the enhanced world view we share. Not all people have an interest in these topics, and it might not be right for you.

You certainly will not agree with everything we cover, and that is purely because of a lifetime of conditioning by your parents, your peers, the media, advertising and maybe even your religion. Many of those beliefs are extremely limiting and are holding you back from reaching the levels we know are easily attainable, without special skills. So, embrace a little discomfort - it is called growing pains.

Equality

All people are not equal. They never have been, and they never will be. Any attempts to make them equal are doomed to failure. Some people are superior to others and they always have been. The vast majority of the world's population are like sheep and they always will be. This is just a plain, simple fact of life. We are not sitting in judgment, just stating the obvious. Not everyone can become healthy, wealthy, powerful and free. The sheep are doomed to mediocrity.

There, you see - we have shocked you a little already! But remember, we have only just begun. As you progress, we intend to stun you a great deal more. This is essential if we are to part the veils of illusion which have prevented all of us from achieving our full potential.

Fresh Wisdom is by its very nature elitist. It is only for the chosen few. People like you who have set foot upon the path of power, freedom, health and wealth. You have chosen that path, and you are to be congratulated!

You may have some doubts at this early stage about what *Fresh Wisdom* actually is. Do not worry - these doubts are normal as one begins this journey of discovery. It will take time for you to understand the various illusions which block the pathway to power and freedom. Much of our material will be concerned with identifying those blocks, helping you to understand them, and finally blowing them away so that you can reach undreamed of levels of health, wealth and power.

Expectations

There are a few points which we should make before you continue. These are important in setting expectations for all of us.

1. We will be discussing Independent Wealth Creation Skills a little later. At no point will you be working for, on behalf of, or for the benefit of Freedom Technology, the publishers of *Fresh Wisdom*. We are not some sort of Multi Level Marketing (MLM) organization.

2. We will be sharing inside information with you, which took many years to accumulate - the hard way. We have chosen to make it available because life-changing information like this should be shared, not kept hidden. The strategies are priceless and are reserved only for *Fresh Wisdom* readers. You will not find this information published anywhere else.

3. The information we will be sharing is in the form of strategies and principles, designed to assist you in living a fulfilled life. This is the kind of information which should have been taught to us at school. We call them Fulfilled Living Principles. How you apply these principles is totally up to you.

4. At certain points we will recommend 'How To' products, which provide further step-by-step guidelines for implementing the strategies discussed. All of the products we recommend support the principles explained. You are under no obligation to purchase any product, and purchasing a particular product does not guarantee success in that area of your life. The only

way you will achieve lasting success in your life is by taking action and implementing what you learn.

5. The people behind *Fresh Wisdom* are contrarian thinkers. We are not legal experts, medical professionals, ministers of religion, investment advisors or licensed counselors. We have purposely not accepted any recognized certification, because we believe this limits the creative thinking required to achieve a truly fulfilled life.

Therefore, it is a condition of your continued reading that you release Freedom Technology from any responsibility for any actions you take as a result of strategies you learn here. By taking any particular course of action discussed in this book, you agree that you are solely responsible for seeking the necessary professional advice before implementing any of the strategies we are going to teach, many of which may be illegal in your country.

There, we believe we have now covered the necessary legal jargon adequately.

In short, we are providing this information because we are frustrated with the lack of truth available today. It is the kind of information we wish we had received earlier in life. And we are sharing it in good faith. It has worked for us, and we fully believe it will work for you. But we cannot guarantee it, and cannot accept responsibility since we do not know your personal circumstances.

4. The Power of a Paradigm

It is important that we understand what a *paradigm* is, and how to make a *paradigm shift*. It is the basis of the entire book and is not as complicated as it may sound.

You may be familiar with the picture below, in which you can see both a young woman and an old woman, in the same picture. If you have seen this before, please do read on – there is an important lesson to be applied.

If you have not seen it before, take a few moments to see if you can identify an elegant woman in her early 20's, and if you focus differently, you will see an old hag.

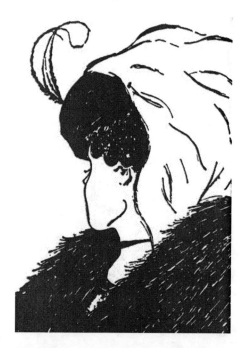

It is important that you can clearly see both women before reading further. If you cannot see both women, go to Appendix A on page 229 for an explanation.

Most people think this is just an interesting party trick. But here is the real value of the picture. An exercise was conducted many years ago at Harvard Business School. The instructor was using it to demonstrate clearly that two people can see the same thing, disagree, and yet both be right. It is not logical, it is psychological.

The instructor handed a set of cards to one half of the class. On it was the following sketch of a young woman.

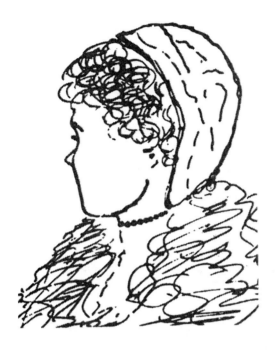

The other half of the class received a card with the following sketch of an old woman.

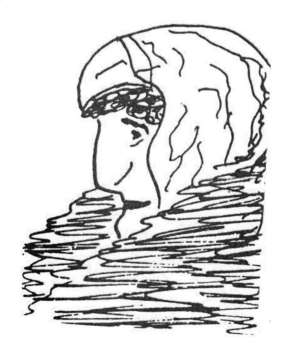

The class was told to concentrate on their cards for 10 seconds, after which the complete picture of both old and young women together was projected onto a screen (the diagram on page 16).

Without exception, those in the class who had seen the picture of the young woman first, could not see the old woman. And vice versa. Only after a considerable period of debate could each group convince the other that there was indeed a picture of the other woman.

Each person in the class could only see what they had been conditioned to see in the initial 10-second period of time.

Conditioning

Why is the result of this exercise so important to us? Well, it shows how powerfully conditioning affects our perceptions, or our paradigms. If ten seconds can have that kind of impact on how we see things, what about the conditioning of a lifetime? The influences in our lives - family, school, church, work environment, friends, associates, and current social conditioning - all have made their silent unconscious impact on us and help shape our frame of reference, our paradigms, the way we see life.

In essence, we have been conditioned to see only the old hag in our general lives. The beauty of the young woman has been kept purposely hidden from us. *Fresh Wisdom* is designed to help you find the young woman hidden in the composite picture of life, so that you can start living a truly Fulfilled Life.

The "Aha!" Experience

Earlier we mentioned a *paradigm shift*. Very simply, it is what we might call the "Aha!" experience, when someone finally sees the slim, attractive young girl when previously all they could see was an old hag. The stronger the initial perception is, the more powerful the "Aha!" experience is. It is as though a light were suddenly turned on inside.

And that is what *Fresh Wisdom* is all about. We are going to show you how many of our perceptions are incorrect, because of conditioning we have all unknowingly been subject to. You are going to experience one "Aha!" experience after another, as we guide you to a fuller understanding of how to live a truly fulfilling life, free of all the previously held limiting beliefs we have been conditioned to accept as truth.

Now, prepare yourself for the next shock.

A Centuries Old Conspiracy

It is far too early in this Seminar to go into all the historical studies
which have proven what we are about to say. You can either take our
word for it or do the research yourself.[2] The fact of the matter is...

...For more than 400 years there has existed a secret and well
coordinated plan to change society's perceptions by conditioning all of
us to believe what *they* want us to believe. *They* have only ever shown
us the picture of the old hag (and it does not necessarily matter who
they are, although you will find hundreds of different theories online[3]).
As a result, most of us cannot see the stunningly beautiful young girl
who is right in front of us, yet invisible. All because of the extent of
our conditioning; this has been passed on for the past 4 or more
generations.

What this means is that all education, all religions, all media,
all forms of government, all medical systems have been purposely
twisted to achieve the conditioning *they* want.

All of the beliefs you currently hold dear have been influenced
by people who do not have your best interests at heart.

- *They* want mega-profits for themselves.
- *They* want to enslave us.
- *They* want us to be unhealthy and fat so that we die at an early age.
- *They* do not want us to think for ourselves.
- *They* want us to spend hours in front of their propaganda machines: TV.
- *They* want us to be limited in our religious beliefs.
- *They* want us to remain poor.
- *They* want us to become miserable failures in the universal scheme of things.

And their dastardly plan is working.[4]

That explains the state of the world currently. And it will become
worse, far worse. Sadly, there is not much we can do about it. The
plan is so far advanced, and so well controlled that there is nothing we
can do to stop it. Resistance is futile.

What Do We Do?

What we can do, though, is rectify our perceptions. Remove the
limiting beliefs which hold us back from achieving all the Creator
wanted us to achieve. But it will not be easy. Changing a lifetime of
perceptions cannot happen overnight. It will take thought, discipline

---

[2] A good place to start is www.ThreeWorldWars.com
[3] www.thewatcherfiles.com/bloodlines/
[4] www.unveilingthem.com/SecretCovenant.htm

and work. It will take a willingness to believe that maybe, just maybe, what we firmly believe right now could well be based on incorrect assumptions. And a willingness to have those assumptions corrected. It will be challenging, but the rewards far outweigh the challenge.

Are you ready for the challenge? Ready to step up to the mark and change your life to one that you just cannot even comprehend right now? You have taken the first step by starting this book. You may well have been shocked by some of the things covered already, and we have plenty more 'positive discomfort' in store for you.

Your Current World View

Very few of the remaining chapters will include exercises, but this is an exception. This will prove a particularly valuable exercise by the time you complete this book, and the sooner you do the exercise, the more effective it will prove.

Start by writing down a list of what you currently believe to be absolutely true, whatever that may be. The more detail you provide, the more powerful the lessons in this book will become. We have suggested a few subject headings, but feel free to add as many as you can think of.

- Love, Relationships and Marriage
- Health, Nutrition and Longevity
- Salaries, Independent Wealth Creation and Money
- Religion and Spirituality
- Personal Freedom, Politics and Democracy

Depending on how thoroughly you completed the exercise, you have just defined your current world view. The important point is this: your world view has been heavily influenced by outside forces that do not have your best interests at heart. This book will challenge your current world view and present an alternative for your careful consideration.

It is not possible to change your fundamental world view overnight. Read the material in this book carefully. There will be much you do not agree with, particularly if you have taken the previous exercise seriously. But by the end of the book you will come to the conclusion that your current paradigm has been purposely conditioned.

5. The Immutable Laws of Nature

The first step to achieving a free and fulfilled life is to understand that all of life is governed by law. This includes Nature, Music, Art and all of the Sciences. Gravity is just such a law. It never changes, and it affects us whether we agree it exists or not.

To live in harmony with the Laws of Nature produces vibrant health, engaging relationships, abundant joy, clarity of thought, unparalleled judgment and a fulfilled life. To violate them produces strife, stress and destruction.

These Laws of Nature are in operation, whether we are aware of them and understand them, or not. And the laws do not 'change with the times' like everything else seems to. The Laws of Nature today are the same Laws of Nature that applied thousands of years ago. They are unchangeable or *immutable*.

Very few of us fully understand the Law of Gravity, and we seldom concern ourselves over it. But it continues working, ensuring a comfortable living environment here on earth. So it is with all the Laws of Nature – unseen yet ever present.

You may already be living a fulfilled life because you understand and abide by these Laws, or you may be trapped in an unfulfilling life because you follow a different set of man-made laws.

Now here's a challenging question...

What Are the Laws of Nature?

Have your parents ever explained them? Did you learn them at school? Does your religion ever mention the Immutable Laws of Nature? In fact, have you ever heard of this term before?

No?

Can you see that maybe, just maybe, important aspects of life have been purposely withheld from us?

It is undeniable that much unnecessary unhappiness exists today because of ignorance of the Immutable Laws of Nature.

Knowledge, understanding and application of these laws lifts our life out of the mediocre and places it on a heavenly plane. It is the flowers rather than the weeds, the banquet rather than the crumbs.

So it would make sense then to discover what these Laws of Nature are, so that we can start following them, and in so doing automatically live a more fulfilling life.

Two-and-a-half millennia ago, Sophocles in his Antigone was the first to recognize the supremacy of Universal Natural Law. Concepts of natural law, rights, and justice subsequently evolved through Socrates, Aristotle, Cicero, Cato, Seneca, the Magna Carta, Aquinas, Sidney, Locke, Adam Smith and John Stuart Mill -- even

Baruch Spinoza with his Universal Man[5] and Immanuel Kant with his Universal Laws[6]. And, finally, Thomas Jefferson climaxed natural law in his Declaration of Independence by recognizing the unalienable rights of each individual to life, liberty, and the pursuit of happiness.

In 51 B.C. Cicero defined Natural Law in *On the Republic*:

"True law is right reason in agreement with nature, universal, consistent, everlasting, whose nature is to advocate duty by prescription and to deter wrongdoing by prohibition. Good men obey its prescriptions and prohibitions, but evil men disobey them.

It is forbidden by God to alter this law, nor is it permissible to repeal any part of it, and it is impossible to abolish the whole of it. Neither the Senate nor the People can absolve us from obeying this law and we do not need to look outside ourselves for an expounder or interpreter of this law.

There will not be one law at Rome and another law at Athens. There is now and will be forever one law, valid for all peoples and all times. And there will be one master and ruler for all of us in common, God, who is the author of this law, its promulgator, and enforcing judge.

Whoever does not obey this law is trying to escape himself and to deny his nature as a human being. By this very fact, he will suffer the greatest penalties, even if he should somehow escape conventional punishments."[7]

The Immutable Laws of Nature have been known since almost the beginning of time, and yet we are no longer taught the importance of these laws.

We will be covering 15 of the most important and relevant to leading a fulfilled life. Following is simply an introduction to the Laws of Nature we will discuss in subsequent chapters.

Relationships

We begin with relationships, since this provides the basic meaning to, and the purpose of life: developing fulfilling relationships. The Laws of Relationships are based on:

- *Dating*: the Law of Attraction - Use this Law to find your ideal partner and avoid falling for the wrong ones.
- *Mating*: the Law of Expectations, or what men and women each want out of a fulfilling relationship.

---

[5] www.yesselman.com/
[6] http://plato.stanford.edu/entries/kant-moral/
[7] *On the Republic* by Cicero (106 BC - 43 BC)
http://sow.colloquium.co.uk/~barrett/cicero.html

- *Ever-Aftering*: the Law of Fidelity between a woman and a man that leads to long-term fulfillment, and how to ensure that your relationship becomes a life long love affair, in which neither partner feels the need to look elsewhere to have their needs fulfilled.

Health & Longevity

Unless you are leading a healthy life, free of dependence on manufactured drugs of any form, your own body will be holding you back from achieving all you can. The Laws of Ultimate Health & Longevity are based on:

- *Taking Responsibility* for one's own health; not becoming dependant on anyone else, including the medical establishment. This requires effort. The first step in taking responsibility is to understand the forces against you: Media; Government; Environment; Health Establishment; Traditions.
- *Natural Lifespan*: Both Science and the Good Book indicate that a normal life-span is 120 years. False information is being used to promulgate the idea that it is only 70 to 80; and that a loss of faculties is inevitable. By changing simple life patterns, achieving a *healthy* life to 120 and even beyond is not only possible, but how the human body was originally designed.

Independent Wealth Creation

Without an independent means of creating wealth, you will forever be a slave to a salaried position. The Laws of Financial Independence & Wealth Creation are based on:

- *Materialization*: This is a fundamental law of the Universe: what the mind of man can conceive, it can bring about. The mind is the workshop in which everything is initially created.
- *Persistence*: Without persistence, very little is ever achieved. With it, anything can be accomplished. Understanding and harnessing it can lead to the achievement of any goal. A plan without persistence is no plan at all.
- *Actualization*: The ultimate reason and purpose for a successful life is to attain transcendent self-actualization. We refer to this as attaining *The Omega Point*. (More about this later.) Self-actualization is to find self-fulfillment and realize one's full potential. The reason this is included under Wealth Creation has to do with the difference between Value Extraction and Value Creation, which we will cover in a subsequent chapter.
- *Leverage*: This law is the principle of taking all of your assets (your time being the most valuable) and making them work for you. Until we can leverage our time, we will never become

wealthy and powerful, and we will never free our time to do the things we enjoy.

Personal Freedom & Independence

Unless we are able to lead a life free of interference from those who want to limit our life, we will never be able to achieve a truly fulfilling life. The Laws of Personal Freedom & Independence are based on:

- *Privacy*: The ongoing erosion of privacy in the World is the most important issue facing individuals today. Without privacy, we have nothing, or less than nothing. Privacy is a human imperative because privacy of self is an important biological necessity of a sane and stable sense of self. It is a scientific fact that a rational person cannot have their autonomous sense of self compromised and still function as a healthy individual.

- *Independence*: Only by having wealth sufficient to free oneself from the shackles of a salaried position, and which you alone control and are aware of, can one achieve a truly fulfilled life. We will provide a mechanism for creating a leveraged, passive income.

- *Sovereignty*: This is the end ideal to be achieved. A king or queen is not only independent, but also leads their people. In fact they *serve* their people. This is the epitome of success, self-actualization and reaching the Omega Point. (We will explain all of this.)

Metaphysical Truths

This may sound a little complex right now, but as you progress through this material all will become clear. Remember that this is simply an introduction. The Laws of Metaphysical Truths are based on:

- *Creation*: The Universe and the mind of man were brought into existence out of nothing - or out of something which is currently beyond the ability of our mind to comprehend - by an Initiator outside of this world system. Once we understand this, our response is usually and almost inevitably, one of awe – not one of rebellion.

- *2 Forces: Positive and Negative.* The positive force is naturally good, and the negative force is naturally evil. The opposing forces were introduced for our personal training. It is how we react to these forces which determine the effectiveness of the training.

These then are the basic Laws of Nature we will be covering in the next few chapters. Do not concern yourself about understanding them all now - this was purely an introduction, and we will be going into far more explanation soon.

Common Violations of the Laws of Nature

The reason we are providing examples of violations of the Laws of Nature is to illustrate the extent to which our lives are limited. We will show you how, by living according to man-made, artificial laws, we often unknowingly limit our ability to live an abundant life.

Relationships

A person not familiar with the Laws of Relationships, engages in the same, identical, mind-stifling routine day after day, year after year. It does not matter what the detail of this routine is, but it might go something like this:

- Come in, kiss your spouse.
- Make cup of coffee or tea.
- Sit down and read paper for half an hour while spouse prepares meal.
- Eat meal, chat about pointless things.
- Argue for a while.
- Wash up.
- Watch television.
- If 2nd Thursday of month, then go to local restaurant.
- Go to bed.
- If 3rd Thursday of month, then make love.
- Go to sleep.
- Repeat until you die.

This may be stereotyped, but the real point is that, married or not, the 'normal' person follows almost exactly the same routines, with very slight variations, every single day, week after week.

Further, attraction is defined by what we see in glossy magazines. In other words, a woman must be slim, tall, pretty and well manicured. A man must be muscular, handsome and well tanned.

Absolute garbage!

Men and women come 'hard-wired' with their own different sets or internal templates of what comprises a desirable mate, and a set of emotional trigger buttons that, when pushed, create that powerful emotional response called *attraction* which compels them to mate with the one who triggers it.

Most have no idea that this mechanism exists or how to trigger it, so they do traditionally 'nice' things which usually have the opposite of the desired effect. Humans do not choose who they feel attraction for, and they do not choose the emotions that they feel either. It just happens - Bam!

What about all the relationship advice that floods our TV screens, magazines and radio stations. All claiming to have THE answer to why more than half of marriages end in divorce.

There are only two vital needs in any relationship. Get this right and everything else falls into place:

- The most important need a man has in a relationship is to feel appreciated, admired and respected. Without his partner's appreciation his life is but an empty shell.
- The most important need a woman has in a relationship is to feel loved and cherished. Without her partner's love her life is but an empty shell.

Without appreciation, there is no love; without love there is no appreciation.

Ever seen that taught anywhere?

It is because the Agony Aunts, Soap Opera Stars and Talk Show Hosts do not understand the Laws of Nature as far as Relationships are concerned, that they violate these Laws, impose their own laws, and in the process create even more unhappiness.

Ultimate Health & Longevity

Here is a little secret about how the medical establishment operates:

- If nature made the cure, you cannot patent it...
- If you cannot patent it, you cannot mark it up for mega-profits...
- And that means you cannot pay for TV commercials, you cannot deluge doctors with samples, you cannot endow universities to bless it with their research, and you cannot afford the legal shenanigans to push it through the FDA.

Almost 93% of non-surgical ailments can be cured effectively by controlling what you put in your mouth from nature. Controlling your food and drink, and enhancing your intake with herbs and supplements.

Nature is the best healer you will ever find, but any breakthroughs as a result of research into natural healing are squashed, before they can affect the profits of all-powerful drug companies.

Drug companies, in their greedy drive for higher profits, have focused on producing drugs which only address the symptoms, often at the expense of worsening the original condition they claim to have been trying to cure. This obviously creates a further profit potential, to sell further drugs to alleviate the additional symptoms. They have violated the Immutable Laws of Nature, imposing their own laws, and in the process have created even more unhappiness and ongoing health problems.

Financial Independence & Wealth Creation

The 'normal' person has barely enough money to live on, because their outgoings either exactly match, or exceed their income, leaving them drifting into debt. In fact the 'normal' person is in debt to a considerable extent, typically owing tens of thousands on a mortgaged home, having finance on one or more expensive items (car, furniture), having a bank overdraft, and owing money on one or more credit cards.

The burden of these debts, together with an 'unchangeable' lifestyle, ensures that Johnny and Jane Average always operate with the tip of their noses *just* above the water. The effect of this is to lock them solidly into the freedom-removing system of salaried work. It prevents them from exploring their full potential and living a joyous life - because they are scared of losing their jobs due to the debts and commitments that weigh them down.

This is not how a fulfilled life is meant to be. Banks, in their greedy drive for higher profits, have made credit increasingly easier to obtain, and in doing so have violated the Immutable Laws of Nature, imposing their own laws, and in the process have created even more unhappiness and slavery.

Personal Freedom & Independence

If you asked any individual living in any Western Democratic Country: "Are you free?" they would almost unhesitatingly reply "Yes, I am free." A few more thoughtful souls might qualify their answer by saying something like: "Yes, I am reasonably free," or "Well, I am as free as anyone else." Most would say that they enjoy a tremendous amount of personal liberty in their private and public lives.

Well, they are all completely wrong. The vast majority of people are about as trapped or 'un-free' as it is possible to get without being manacled to the wall of some dank cell.

They have almost no freedom in any area of their lives. They have allowed themselves to be absolutely and rigorously controlled by outside forces - other people - to the extent that they can barely shuffle around and make grunting noises through their gags. Only those who have correctly understood and applied the principles of Personal Freedom & Independence can be said to be truly free. The rest are, to a greater or lesser extent, slaves.

Consider this:

The 'normal' person works for a living in a job which they either actively dislike, or just tolerate. A few 'lucky' souls occasionally enjoy some aspects of their job - on a good day. The 'normal' person has to get to work at a certain time every single day of the working week. They dare not be late or leave before a certain time, under threat of some form of penalty.

Thus, approximately forty hours of every single week - week in, week out - are governed and ruled by the dictates of someone else. No matter how liberal the company, no matter how nice the boss, no matter how much flexi-time is offered, the stark truth is that for about forty hours every week, the 'normal' person hands over complete control of their life to other people, who make them sing and dance more or less like a puppet.

Here is something else:

The 'normal' person willingly hands over at least *fifty percent* of their personal wealth, in the form of taxes, to other people to spend as they see fit. They neither ask for, nor expect accountability. They do not know where their money is spent (except in the vaguest way), and they do not care. They do not ask for facts and figures, or expect accountability, honesty or efficiency. If they try to withhold their money, then agents of force come and take them away and throw them in jail. They accept this as reasonable and normal.

They are taught nothing whatsoever in school about how their own government handles the country's finances. If they were to ask the government for an itemized bill of where their money (taxes) had been spent, they would be met with blank stares and vague answers. But we are not finished yet!

The 'normal' person reads newspapers, watches television news and current affairs, listens to radio news broadcasts and actually *believes* many of the items they hear.

More importantly, they spend a significant amount of their time *debating* these issues with friends, and pontificating about the rights and wrongs of the particular issue in question. In this manner, their emotions are controlled by whatever news story the media decide they will release to them that day. They hold a huge collection of *opinions* and *views* about every conceivable topic from nuclear power to abortion, and spend a significant amount of their time explaining and defending these views.

This, despite the fact that they often have almost no knowledge at all about these topics, and are merely repeating 'information bites' released by the media.

They watch televised debates about a certain topical issue, and actually take one side or another – even to the extent of becoming hot under the collar when the opposition view is being expressed. In this way, their opinions and views are safely polarized into one camp or another, and firmly away from any *real* choices, decisions or debates.

So it is clear that no-one living in any Western democracy is in fact free. We are *all* bound by extremely limiting beliefs and lifestyles.

Metaphysical Truths

The 'normal' person believes, either overtly, or covertly, that there is some sort of all-powerful god or supernatural being, watching over them. This same being has a kind of book, in which it marks the times when you have been a good boy or girl, and the times when you have been a naughty boy or girl. When you die, if the good points do not outweigh the naughty points then you will be severely punished - possibly for all eternity. So the 'normal' person struggles all of their life to try and live by rules imposed by other people, or groups of people, or warped religions. They worry if laws are transgressed, and they spend a certain amount of time agonizing, looking over their shoulders or confessing their 'sins'.

Even those who profess atheism still retain a nagging doubt in the back of their minds that somewhere a score is being kept of their good deeds vs. their bad deeds. There are very, very few people who are free of this man-made belief.

The vast majority of religions are wrong. The meaning of the original teachings of the world's major religions have been twisted, altered and decimated by those looking to benefit either financially or egotistically. Individual religious leaders have violated the Immutable Laws of Nature, imposing their own laws, and in the process have created even more unhappiness.

~~~

We realize that the situations described above could not possibly apply to you, but we mention them purely as examples of modern day violations of the Immutable Laws of Nature.

It is undeniable that much unnecessary unhappiness exists today because of ignorance or violation of the Immutable Laws of Nature.

This book will teach you the Laws of Nature, and show you with empirical proof how living within the minor confines of these laws will lead to a fulfilled life.

If you are feeling uneasy at this point with any of the material we have covered, perhaps we can reassure you with the following statement: -

A strong, wealthy, powerful and free person is far, far better equipped to really help someone, or to improve a bad situation, than a weak, pathetic, poor and trapped sheep.

By the end of this book you will be able to move into every situation with *power* and *true integrity*. You will bring about real and lasting changes in your own life, and in the lives of those around you. Just being near you will be enough for others to see and feel your very real power. Let us see where this little journey might lead.

6. How Media Molds Our Minds

By media we mean radio, television, newspapers, magazines, films, billboard advertising, books and junk mail; to mention only a few. We truly do live in an environment in which information is power, which means that information is also money. A great many companies are now dedicated purely to accumulating, processing and selling information and this situation is increasing almost exponentially. The more channels there are available for the distribution of information (cable TV, satellite TV, video, new radio channels, the Internet, etc.) the more companies proliferate to exploit the desire of the sheep for all this information.

The Information Age

We live in a society where information abounds: Radio, television, newspapers, magazines, periodicals, the Internet and other electronic media, satellite communications, and all manner of religions and governments. However, the information age does not equal the age of truth. Increasing information does not necessarily mean a greater understanding of reality.

Today's society is not led by a zeal for honesty, but rather by powerful economic and socio-political forces bent on maintaining whatever status quo suits them.

Those in power generally use unscrupulous methods to remain there, and likewise with the economically powerful, who frequently use fraudulent means to maintain their positions.

Today, ideas compete for money and power more than ever before. Integrity is usually never even considered.

The Media Con

Media operators attempt to con values from you under false pretences. The values they seek are primarily money, and secondarily influence. They are con-artists because they are more often than not secretive about their motives. Instead, the media masquerade as altruistic champions of the people, fighting the corner for their readers/viewers and facing every danger to selflessly bring the latest important news story from far-flung corners of the globe.

The pay-off for the media is money, power and influence. The pay-off for the sheep is the rather sad and pathetic belief that they actually know what is going on around the world - when they do not; and a feeling that, because they understand the 'latest issues', they have personal power - which they do not.

The media operate by selectively presenting you with edited snippets of world news. These snippets are the pieces which they believe you will be most interested in. And most of the time, they are selected purely for their degree of sensationalism, because this is what sells.

Using these 'news' items, the media attempt to manipulate your emotions in order to get you to feel what they think you should feel. They also offer opinions which they attempt to get you to subscribe to. Even up-market newspapers present an extremely narrow cross-section of current world news. A few stories are selected from thousands of possible stories by the editor. His or her job is to present you with a version of reality which he or she thinks you will find most acceptable. By 'acceptable' we mean that you will be willing to pay good money to purchase that particular version of reality.

Newspapers exist to make profit for their already wealthy owners. Pure and simple. Some of the most wealthy and powerful men in the world today are media tycoons[8]. It is your purchase of their newspapers and magazines that made them so extraordinarily wealthy.

This is the only reason they exist. Dismiss from your mind any notion that newspapers exist as a kind of public-spirited information service which altruistically keeps the citizens informed of the latest important world events.

How Does the Media Make Money?

They make their money mainly through selling advertising space or air time. They also make money on the cover price of the paper or magazine. This is their prime concern - how to sell as much top priced advertising space as possible.

From this, it follows that the bigger the circulation of your newspaper/magazine, or the more people who watch your TV program (and hence the adverts during the commercial breaks), the more you can charge for advertising. Indeed, this is exactly the case. The amount you pay for advertising is directly related to the number of potential punters you are going to reach. This means that the publications are forever striving to increase their circulations.

How do you increase your circulation? Certainly not by printing hard facts about various global events. They sell more copies by playing on your emotions to extract your hard earned cash. Headlines like: *"Naked Clergy in Sex Romp Shock"* sells far more papers than: *"US Car Production Efficiency Up By 11%"*, although the latter news item is likely to have far more effect on the reader's life than the former.

The most effective way of increasing circulation is to print stories which play on emotions: fear, guilt, etc.

---

[8] www.cjr.org/tools/owners/

People read these stories, believe them, and instantly make the 'facts' of the story into their own 'considered' opinion.

For the duration of the 'hot' story (rarely longer than three days unless thousands of lives are affected), they will then discuss and debate with friends, family and anyone else who will listen. During these discussions, they will regurgitate the news exactly as received by them from the media.

This gives them the pay-off of feeling powerful (because they think they know all about the latest issues, and have strong opinions about them). It also makes them feel caring (because they can start the conversation with "Isn't it awful about...", or "Did you hear that terrible story about..."). It also reduces their guilt because they believe that by knowing about a problem, and discussing it, they are somehow reducing it.

These people are truly powerless, because they are doing absolutely nothing about the news item. All their talk, debating and pontificating has absolutely zero effect on the event itself.

These people are also ignorant, because they know almost nothing about the true situation. They know only a handful of opinions, lies and sensationalist garbage printed by the newspapers. These they call 'facts', and rapidly change them into their own 'considered opinions'. These people are also uncaring hypocrites because they choose to debate instead of actually doing something to help.

How to Read the News

The *Fresh Thinker* has a better idea of how to handle the world's media. We know how to respond to news articles on, for example, disasters. We rarely read them because they are such gross distortions of the truth.

Most of the time, if the article does not affect our life directly, we choose to do nothing about it. We realize that we cannot actually care about people in far-flung corners of the earth. We also realize the selective nature of these stories. For every disaster which makes the front page, there are several thousand which will never be mentioned because they are not sufficiently sensational.

We have absolutely no opinion whatsoever on these stories. Accordingly we will never become involved in a discussion about the latest disaster. The reason we have no opinion is because we know that we have little direct knowledge of the facts, and the story does not affect our life directly.

While the sheep are feeling sad, guilty and filled with doom, we are getting on with our life, and feeling good, happy and fulfilled.

This is the most important point. The sheep do nothing about the disaster and then waste their time feeling sad and guilty, or pontificating, debating, arguing and waffling about the subject to the other sheep. We too do nothing about the disaster and then we spend our time in happy, guilt-free, life-enhancing pursuits.

We know that the media circus exists to make money and not to provide reliable, accurate information. If they can get the story roughly accurate, they will print something which approximates reality. But if they are short of facts, or the story needs a little more spice, then they will invent the missing pieces.

This is particularly true of the tabloids.

It therefore follows, does it not, that it would be illogical, even foolish to act on the basis of a newspaper story - for example, to give money away to an appeal.

It is also foolish to waste a second of your precious life in debating or discussing newspaper stories. You might just as well spend an evening debating whether Jack or the Giant was the real baddie in the story of *Jack and the Beanstalk*. After all, Jack did invade the Giant's home and stole his gold, his harp and his hen. We ought to have a phone-in on this subject so that we can all debate this important issue - on air!

Are Reputable Newspapers Also Guilty?

The more reputable papers try to resist the temptation to blatantly invent the facts, but they still suffer from the 'lie' of editing. That is, a certain story presented in the quality press might be approximately correct in its rough outline, but why was that particular story selected, and a hundred other stories ignored?

The reason is that the editor believes that you will be more interested in the story he has selected for you, than all the others. He has made up your mind for you on this, and you will not be consulted. You will also not even get a glimpse of the other stories. They might as well never have happened.

Just the same as we would never allow someone else to decide which novel we should read, or what music we will listen to, or which restaurant we will enjoy dinner in, so we refuse to have someone else decide which news articles are relevant and important. To remain abreast of current events we choose instead independent publications[9], and are willing to pay a higher price for more accurate and complete reporting.

Global Media Control

There is a far more sinister reason for the editing of news on a global basis. It is not only individual newspaper editors who filter news

---

[9] www.freedomtechnology.org/resources/altmedia.htm

information. If that were the case, we would receive a healthy variety of opinions between the various tabloids.

The situation is far worse than that. There are presently only 3 major news agencies, all owned and controlled by media moguls who are fully aligned with the plan to introduce a Global Government. These moguls receive vast government handouts to carefully control and manipulate public opinion by what is printed and aired on television. This explains why all the news conforms to a narrow agenda. Try flicking stations between CNN and BBC during the coverage of a newsworthy event – the commentary and coverage are almost identical.

An excellent exposé of how news events are manipulated by Hollywood style directors can be seen in the movie *Wag the Dog* with Dustin Hoffman.

Incidentally, have you ever been on an international holiday, or been away from your home country for two or more weeks? On your return you realize that you have not heard any news for two weeks. All of those stories have been born, risen to prominent attention, and then died again. Phone-ins have discussed the stories, current affairs programs have waffled on about the stories, and you missed all of it. Are you a poorer person for having missed any of it? Do you feel that there is a huge gap in your knowledge? Did you worry about any of these stories that you missed? Of course not! Why? Because you were enjoying yourself and living a fulfilled life. You were far too busy having a great time to worry about all that nonsense going on back home.

Phone-Ins, Opinion Polls and Letters to the Editor

Phone-in programs are further classic examples of weak and powerless people struggling for a modicum of approval from other people (again, total strangers).

Phone-in programs almost always deal with the latest media issue of the day. As we have already explained, these issues are largely artificial, transitory and of no consequence. Yet the sheep get hot under the collar. They become desperate to join in the debate, to make their point, to have other people hear their views on the subject. And, of course, each caller knows that their viewpoint is the only valid viewpoint and that the other callers must be crazy to take any opposing view.

The people who take part in these programs rarely have an informed opinion on the subject. Instead, they are simply regurgitating back to the media, snippets of sheep fodder handed out to them earlier by the self-same media. People telephone these programs because they hold a rag-bag collection of opinions on every subject under the sun.

No matter what the issue, they can drag out an opinion to suit - and they cannot wait until the rest of the nation has heard it.

The participants are desperately seeking a little bit of personal power for themselves. They revel in the feeling that the whole nation has heard their prejudices and biased version of reality. They can bask in the warm glow of achievement for months after the show. The truth is, of course, that there are two types of people who listen to these shows:

Those who listen to have a laugh at the arrogant, self-opinionated and often downright ridiculous people who phone in.

Those who listen merely to baa "Quite correct!" after hearing one caller, and "Garbage!" after hearing another caller with the opposite view.

Phone-ins encourage the sheep to stampede for pen A or pen B (follow a particular, pre-determined line of thinking). Once herded into their pens, they are encouraged to 'baa' angrily at the sheep in the opposite pen. The media circus keeps this whole charade going for exactly the run-time of the program, and then cuts it dead. After a day or two, the entire issue will be dropped by the media, in favor of another, equally trivial, but 'hot' issue.

Television, Video, Films

So far we have concentrated mainly on newspapers in this release, but many of the comments apply to all of the media. It is an amazing fact that only eighty years ago, there was no television, no radio. There was also little cinema to speak of. The only media were the newspapers.

Go back another hundred years and newspapers hardly existed. There would be the odd crudely printed sheet of paper carrying some particular piece of news. There were also books, but most people were illiterate, and books were completely out of the financial league of the common people - apart from the Bible.

Media is a very modem phenomenon. People living in the 1700's and earlier would rarely have heard anything about anything. They would know what was going on in the next village. They would hear once a week a few facts about the next town, and they would hear every few months, a few facts about other countries - but that would be it.

Nowadays, we are bombarded day and night by a constant stream of media output, most of it aimed at trying to alter your life from what you want it to be, to what they want it to be. The most obvious of these techniques is advertising. Most advertisers are selling image first, and product second. In other words they are trying to get you to aspire towards being something different. Notice all TV car adverts. Very few explain the features and benefits of the car – instead they focus solely on the image you will project by owning the car.

How Should We Handle the Media?

A *Fresh Thinker* will listen to the news on TV or radio roughly once every other day, purely to keep abreast of what is going on.

We never buy newspapers or magazines.

We watch TV for no more than two hours per week. This would be an educational program of interest, or an occasional entertainment program. The reason for this low viewing time is that we have more important life-enhancing things to do than watching television. Watching TV is the ultimate vegetable occupation. Agreed, it is nice just to slump in an armchair sometimes, but we are far more likely to do this with a book, rather than gawping at a screen.

Please understand that we are not attempting to dictate your viewing habits. The point is that television and videos and films and adverts are all trying to interfere with your own perceptions of what you are, and where you are going. Adverts do this by making you aspire towards a lifestyle. Many films deal purely in stereotypes. This makes men want to be Rambo or Clint Eastwood. It makes women believe that 'romantic happy ever after love' exists, and is even normal. It makes all of us believe that extreme violence is normal, and that victims get up and walk away.

We do not want to labor these points too much. It is enough to say that media output (including films and videos) deal in illusions. Although it is nice to be told a story sometimes, there is a very great danger that if you are swamped by it night and day, you will be unable to distinguish illusion from reality. Most people are like this already. You are NOT 'most people'. You are attempting to gain firm and powerful control over your life. This means that you will inevitably start acting and thinking differently from those around you. If they watch five hours of soap operas a week, then they earn your pity. If they sit in front of the box for fifteen hours a week (the national average!) then they earn your contempt and pity. Imagine: fifteen whole hours a week. Just think what you could do with that time!

Why the Media Obsession?

One of the reasons that people allow themselves to fill their lives with all these distractions is because they really, truly do not have anything more important to do. If we were to free these people from the need to work (say by paying the equivalent of their salary) they would be completely at a loss. And that is not temporarily, we mean permanently. They really do not have anything much that they want to do with their lives. It is true - they would not watch TV for fifteen hours a week if they had things they really wanted to do.

This single fact is what distinguishes you and us from ordinary people. We have things - dozens of things - which we want to do with our lives. If we had ten more lifetimes, we would cram them full. We are almost like people who have been given six months to live. If you were given six months to live, would you spend most of it watching TV? Of course not. There is little point in grasping personal freedom if you panic at the thought of being free. There is a penalty to becoming free. Suddenly, the game is up. You have to face yourself and decide what you want to do with what little remains of your life. It is scary, but fun. You and us have a whole long list of things we want to do, from learning the piano to climbing Mount Everest. Normal people, in contrast, have little or nothing they want to do. Given the opportunity, they would stare at you blankly and come up with....nothing.

This reason alone is why most people allow themselves to be controlled by the illusions. They collude in the control. They want to be controlled because they are terrified of examining their lives and finding that the cupboard is bare.

~~~

At this stage of this journey, we want you to start taking a good, long, hard, honest look at yourself. Are there things you really want to do? Are you aware that once you become free, you will actually be able to do these things? Have you used your lack of freedom as an excuse for not starting the things you claim you want to do? Is the cupboard bare, or do you have untapped depths of creativity within you? These are tough questions, but we want you to answer them for yourself. You cannot *buy* freedom and power, you have to truly want it, and work at it yourself. We can show you the way, but you have to really want to walk down the path we are pointing out to you.

7. Fascinating Relationships

Let us begin with an extremely controversial statement:
If you are currently, or have been in the past:
- Married to, or living with a partner; or
- Engaged to, or seriously involved with a partner,

then you have been exposed to the most dangerous con facing anyone trying to achieve a fulfilled relationship.

That is correct: marriage and engagement, in the way commonly understood by the masses, is the biggest con ever perpetrated on the human race since the start of modern history.

Now we fully expect you to have some difficulty in accepting a statement like this, but we did warn you at the beginning of this Life Manual that you would not find all of the material we cover palatable.

The Wrong Reasons to Start a Relationship

So let us take some time to show you that relationships in this modern day and age come about by pure fluke, or randomly, and these same random reasons are then used to start a lifetime commitment together, including getting married. Here are some of the common reasons people 'fall in love', and ultimately end in marriage:
- They just drift into relationships. This represents just another uncontrolled and random area of their lives;
- They believe in the myth of 'happy ever after love' and believe that marriage is one way of securing that myth;
- They want sex, and a committed relationship is the only way they know of getting it;
- Their sexual (and biological) desires override their logic and make them think that they are 'in love';
- They want a replacement figure (e.g. Mother, Father);
- They allow their age to influence their decision, e.g. they think it is about time that they settled down;
- They allow others (e.g. parents or peers) to pressurize them into getting married, engaged or even start dating;
- They are just plain scared of being left alone, and out of fear become desperate for a relationship.

If you are currently in a committed relationship, can you identify the reason you started that relationship? Can you identify the reason your partner started? Come on, be honest with yourself – it is only you and us going through this right now. Go back and read the list again, and be honest with yourself.

The Right Reason to Start a Relationship

Now, in stark contrast to this collection of ludicrous reasons, *Fresh Thinkers* enter into relationships for one reason only:

A fulfilled relationship commences when both partners believe that the mutual and honest exchange of each other's contribution to the relationship will lead to a temporary increase in happiness for both partners.

Notice the word *temporary* in the above statement.

For a truly free and happy individual, relationships (both platonic and romantic) are always temporary. We do not expect a relationship to last beyond its allotted span, and we know that any attempt to force the relationship to go beyond its natural time-limit would result in unhappiness for both people in the relationship.

This is not a depressing thought at all. In fact exactly the opposite. We have a wonderful, joyous, life-enhancing relationship with our partner, and then may move on to the next different, equally wonderful relationship with a different partner. In this way our life is one of constant growth and development, instead of boredom and stagnation.

Notice we are not suggesting for a minute that it makes sense to have a number of simultaneous 'flings', always on the look-out for someone a little better than the current partner. We *are* suggesting that you simply refuse to stay in a relationship which has ended.

When has a Relationship Ended?

A relationship has ended when either:
- there is no longer a mutual and honest exchange of contribution, or
- the initial increase in happiness for both partners has completely disappeared.

When either or both of the situations above come about, it no longer makes sense for the relationship to continue. Going to marital counseling, crying about it, begging your partner for another chance, or demanding that they change to suit your desires, praying to God to save your marriage, or any of the other crazy things we do when a relationship has ended, *does not address the core issue*. It may delay the inevitable, but it cannot recreate the increase in happiness. And if you are not constantly increasing happiness, (apart from the occasional rocky patches in which the strength of each person's commitment is tested), why continue with the relationship?

It is worth pointing out at this point that we are not saying that all relationships *must* be temporary. In fact, later on we are going to show you strategies which virtually guarantee a Life-Long Love Affair. But it is very important that you understand this basic principle:

Expecting a relationship to last forever because your religion says it must, or because that is what you want, or because that is what you have been brought up to believe, is the saddest con anyone can ever fall prey to.

It is probably necessary to back up a little here and answer a few questions for the sake of clarity. Before we do, if you remember back to one of our first lessons, we are in the process of creating "Aha!" moments - moments where we finally understand *why* things may have gone wrong in the past, and what we can do to improve things in the future.

We are not convincing you to accept that your life will necessarily become an endless series of short, meaningless flings.

We are trying to point out that when expectations and perceptions are incorrect from the start, the basis of any relationship is already flawed, and building a Life-Long Love Affair on flawed principles is bound to fail.

To show you how ludicrous the expectation is that a marriage is for life, let us look at some examples from non-romantic relationships.

Platonic Friendships

Have you ever said to a new friend: "I enjoy your company and I think we have a lot in common. I would like for our friendship to develop, but I need some sort of commitment from you that the time and energy I invest in you will not be wasted. So I have drawn up this little agreement which basically promises that you will be my friend until one of us dies."?

You have never said that to a friend? Good! So why on earth would you want to say that to someone you are proposing marriage to?

Friendships are typically allowed to run their course without the constraints of any contract. When either or both friends decide that there is no longer a mutual and honest exchange of contributions, the friendship ends.

Business Agreements

When two or more partners start a new business together, one of the first things they consider is the framework within which the business will operate. This is usually formalized in a contract, which covers all of the terms and conditions necessary for an effective business partnership. Nothing surprising there.

However, an important part of these contracts is planning for failure. That is correct, business people are sensible enough to realize that it is naive to expect a business relationship to last forever, and so draw up guidelines at the beginning for what to do when the business should dissolve.

Even in business agreements, which often involve significant investment in time and capital, there is never an expectation that the relationship will last forever.

So why have the expectation in marriage?

Marriage Contracts

Before a couple get married, it is common to sign some sort of agreement in which both parties state how they would like to share their possessions. The oldest form of contract is where the union takes place in community of property. This is the default method because you do not have to do anything other than arrive at the place of marriage on the right day at the correct time.

More recently, a more formalized contract has been defined: The Ante Nuptial Contract. (Ante = before. Nuptial = marriage. Contract = Bondage). To complicate matters, the ANC (Ante Nuptial Contract) can be with, or without, Accrual.

We are not going to discuss the meaning of each type of contract, but we must make the following point:

By signing *any* of those agreements, you are planning for failure. Every single one of those contracts are agreements on what will happen to your joint possessions when the marriage fails.

So the obvious question is "If a newly married couple (and all the people around them telling them they will live happily ever after) expect their marriage to last forever, why *start* the relationship with an agreement on what to do when it *ends*?"

Are you beginning to see how much of a con this whole "marriage for life" thing is?

The Evidence of Statistics

Statistics in most Western nations show that currently, 2 out of every 3 marriages end in divorce. Despite this commonly-known fact, most people still enter marriage with the idea that it is going to last forever. The statistics are proving what we already know - only, most people are too afraid to admit it. They would rather put their heads in the sand and believe a lie than face up to the truth.

Why Do the Uneducated Expect Lifelong Marriages?

The main reason most people expect marriages to be for life is because of religious teachings. This is true whether you are religious or not. In recent history religious institutions, particularly the church, have played an important role in shaping our core beliefs and life systems. While we will not discuss any particular religion in this section, we do want to make another controversial statement:

- A religion is a system invented by an elite priesthood who desire to extricate value from their followers.

We go to great lengths to prove the accuracy of this statement in a future chapter on Metaphysical Truths.

Fear is probably the major weapon used by religious con-artists over the centuries. As a priest, what better method could you devise for controlling the masses than to pretend that you have a direct line to God, and that He had given you detailed instructions about how other people should behave? If they do not dance to your tune, then you can threaten them with everlasting damnation.

Needless to say, religious teachings on the matter of divorce have caused countless marriages to endure a seemingly endless hell on earth, purely because the couple is too scared to accept that their relationship has reached a natural end. Their church has taught them that divorce is wrong and that they should stick it out.

Without getting ahead of ourselves, this teaching on divorce is certainly not Biblical. We will be covering this in a future chapter.

Open, Honest Relationships

When you understand and embrace the concept that *all* things in nature are temporary, you are able to enjoy guilt-free, honest, open, loving, non-manipulative relationships with your partner. Why should we think completely contrary to nature in only this one area of our lives? It is further proof of the con that we have been led to believe. Fascinating relationships will last exactly as long as they last, and will end when one or both partners cease to enhance the other's life values; or it will end when one or both partners start to inhibit, destroy or harm the other's life values.

A vital point to understand is that in a relationship like this you are 100% honest with your partner. You would never promise to stay 'until death do us part'. You *will* promise to stay until such a time that you cease to bring fulfillment to each other. You *might* promise to do everything in your power to increase the level of fulfillment and enhance your partner's life values, for as long as you are alive.

In contrast, most sheep are con-artists because they promise that they will stay with their partners forever, come what may. This is either an outright lie, because they realize (or suspect) that this is a wholly unachievable fantasy, and that there is only a tiny chance that it will work out this way; or simply a very naïve outlook on life. Again, look at divorce statistics all over the world.

We have been uncharacteristically negative in this chapter, and we have done this intentionally to change your perceptions of what a marriage and lifelong love affair should be. All we urge you to do, is to think about these things in an open and honest manner, with the will to sincerely seek the truth and to no longer be blinded by lies, no matter how painful this process may be. We guarantee that as the shackles fall away, your life will change in miraculous ways and you will become a happier, more fulfilled and enlightened human being.

Now that we have established correct principles for a relationship we can move on to the far more positive aspects of building a truly fulfilling relationship.

In the next Fascinating Relationships chapter we will be covering strategies for turning your romantic relationship into a Life-Long Love Affair.

~~~

Love at first sight is easy to understand; it's when two people have been looking at each other for a lifetime that it becomes a miracle. – Amy Bloom

Love never dies a natural death. It dies because we don't know how to replenish its source. It dies of blindness and errors and betrayals. It dies of illness and wounds; it dies of weariness, of witherings, of tarnishings. – Amais Nin

Love is patient, love is kind.
It does not envy, it does not boast, it is not proud.
It is not rude, it is not self-seeking.
It is not easily angered, it keeps no record of wrongs.
Love does not delight in evil, but rejoices with the truth.
It always protects, always trusts, always hopes, always perseveres.
Love never fails. - I Corinthians 13:4-8

For there is one thing I can safely say: that those bound by love must obey each other if they are to keep company long. Love will not be constrained by mastery; when mastery comes, the God of love at once beats his wings, and farewell -- he is gone. Love is a thing as free as any spirit; women naturally desire liberty, and not to be constrained like slaves; and so do men, if I shall tell the truth. - Chaucer

When we understand that man is the only animal who must create meaning, who must open a wedge into neutral nature, we already understand the essence of love. Love is the problem of an animal who must find life, create a dialogue with nature in order to experience his own being. – Ernest Becker

43

8. Ultimate Health & Longevity

It seems everywhere one turns today, there is so much conflicting advice regarding health. And wherever you turn, there is someone shouting at you:

- You are not eating enough *vegetables!*
- You are not getting enough *exercise!*
- Give up *meat!*
- Give up *coffee!*
- Get out of the *sun!*
- While you are at it, *give up everything!*

But even though everyone else is giving up coffee, alcohol, meat, eggs, fatty foods, sunshine and all the things that used to make life enjoyable... Even though they are exercising like maniacs, sweating like horses, starving themselves on the latest fad diet and scolding you for not joining them... Please do not submit to this self-denial because...

It is just *junk medicine*, and could well be doing your long-term health more harm than good. It may look and sound like the real thing, but when you see what many of these commonly held health and medical beliefs actually do to you, you will be appalled.

While the masses meekly submit to these pseudo-science sacred cows, not even your doctor dares to ask, Why? How come? Says who?

But we are going to ask all those questions right now and you will love the *real answers*, as we break through the myths and cons the medical establishment and health industries have foisted on us, all in the name of higher profits for themselves.

The last thing the medical establishment (perhaps not your doctor personally) wants from you is good health.

The last thing the diet industry wants from you is to lose weight.

Both are in the game purely for money. Neither have your interests at heart, and both will tell you as many lies as possible so that they can extract as much money as possible from you.

Remember this simple truth which drives both the medical establishment and the diet industry:

- If nature made the cure, you cannot patent it.
- If you cannot patent it, you cannot mark it up for mega-profits.

That is the simple reason doctors no longer prescribe natural herbs. It is the simple reason diet programs always promote their formulas instead of fresh, natural, healthy fruit and vegetables:

There is no money in it!

Be Honest With Yourself

Even before getting into the meat of this chapter, ask yourself the following questions. And be honest with yourself - your life is at stake.

- When visiting a doctor, do you want to heal yourself, or are you willing to simply pay someone else to accept responsibility for your health and recovery?
- When you start a diet, are you doing it to improve your overall health, or are you hoping for the quick weight loss the slick sales copy promised?

Depending on your honest answer, the common approach is to simply throw money at a problem instead of tackling the problem head on. The medical establishment and diet industry realize that people are searching for quick-fix answers and capitalize on this for immense profits.

The masses have become overly dependent on their local doctor. This is because of conditioning by the media, government programs, the medical establishment and tradition. However, the typical treatment nowadays is anything which suppresses the symptoms, thus creating the illusion of curing the patient.

Treating the Symptom Instead of the Cause

The body only becomes ill to eradicate or overcome whatever it is that may be throwing the body out of equilibrium. To fast-track the process by means of say, treating the fever as opposed to treating the cause of the fever, results in whatever caused the fever to remain in the body. After a short while it will regroup and recruit more backup before attacking the system once again. Each attack is done with more strength and vigor.

The result is that the patient keeps returning to the doctor who once again treats the disease and not the cause, and a build-up of poisons in the body commences. Of course, doctors are pleased with this outcome because it means more prescriptions of expensive drugs, which translate into more profits.

So, doctors do not in fact promote wellness and health. They simply prolong the inevitable and are to a degree responsible for many build-ups within their patients that result in acute sickness and disease in the long run.

One need just look around to see how many people are suffering from lifestyle diseases such as cancer, diabetes, osteoporosis, arthritis, and allergies, despite regular visits to their doctor. All of these diseases can be controlled and in many cases cured by simply changing whatever is placed in the mouth.

Health Misperceptions

Here are two common health misperceptions, chosen purely as examples of common erroneous beliefs.

Coffee

Contrary to popular belief, coffee (fresh ground organic beans, not instant coffee which is full of contaminants, coloring agents, industrial solvents, and more) is one of nature's real health miracles.

- 1-3 cups of coffee a day reduces the chance of suffering from gallstones by up to 45%
- Have 4 cups a day and you dramatically reduce your risk of colon cancer (the second deadliest cancer in the Western world)
- Just one cup of coffee a day packs the antioxidant power of three fresh oranges.

Still think carefully chosen coffee is bad for you?

Sunshine

You have heard it before: *Sunshine Causes Melanoma.* Just the opposite, in fact. In studies all over the world, as sun exposure increases, malignant skin cancer risk decreases. In the sunniest parts of Australia, lifeguards have lower skin cancer rates than office workers.

In fact, sunshine directly onto our skin and into the retina of the eyes (indirectly) is essential for good health. The key is to never, ever burn your skin. You have to start slowly (15 minutes a day, before 11am or after 3pm); then you can build up to an hour a day or more, depending on your skin type.

So go on out and enjoy the sun sensibly.

The Immutable Laws of Nature Regarding Health

Let us remind ourselves which of the Immutable Laws of Nature which apply to Health and Longevity we are going to discuss.

- *Taking responsibility* for one's own health; not becoming dependent on anyone else, including the medical establishment. This requires effort. The first step in taking responsibility is to understand the forces against you: Media; Government; Environment; Health Establishment; Traditions.
- *Natural lifespan*: Both science and the Good Book indicate that a normal life-span is 120 years. False information is being used to promulgate the idea that it is only 70 to 80; and that a loss of faculties is inevitable. By changing simple life patterns, achieving a healthy life to 120 and even beyond is not only possible, but how the human body was originally designed.

Taking Responsibility for One's Own Health

The most important aspect of taking responsibility for one's health is an understanding and acceptance of the role food plays in your general health and well-being. Everything that passes your lips is either detrimental to or beneficial to your health. There is no such thing as a food that does not affect your health.

San Ssu-Mo, a Taoist physician who correctly diagnosed and cured the nutritional-deficiency disease beriberi 1,300 years ago, a full millennium before European doctors did in 1642, wrote this:

> *"A truly good physician first finds out the cause of the illness, and having found that, he first tries to cure it with food. Only when food fails does he prescribe medication."* [10]

Not quite the same as modern medicine, is it? Of course, the simple reason is that there is a higher profit margin in prescription medicines than in food.

Dr. Charles Mayo, one of the most celebrated American physicians of the 20th Century, said this:

> *"Normal resistance to disease is directly dependent upon adequate nutrition. Normal resistance to disease never comes out of pill boxes. Adequate nutrition is the cradle of normal resistance, the playground of normal immunity, the workshop of good health, and the laboratory of long life."* [11]

The six major causes of premature death in any Western society have all been linked to dietary factors: heart disease, cancer, strokes, diabetes, arteriosclerosis, and cirrhosis of the liver.

It is clear then that a major change in Western dietary habits would have a powerful preventative impact on these deadly diseases. And it would severely impact the lucrative medical, pharmaceutical and food processing industries. This would explain the findings of a Federal Research Committee in 1985: American medical schools do not provide physicians with even the most rudimentary education in nutritional therapy, despite a growing awareness of the role food plays in health and well-being.

So, already you can see that taking responsibility of your own health is as simple as eating sensibly. The challenge is that the understanding of 'eating sensibly' has been so distorted by the results of research funded by mega-corporations, that for most people it has become impossible to know, with absolute certainty, which foods have the most beneficial impact on one's health. In the next Health chapter we will cover what it really means to eat sensibly. And it is not nearly as complicated as you would think.

---

[10] San Ssu-mo, Tang Dynasty (618-907AD)

[11] Dr. Charles H. Mayo, M.D., famed physician, surgeon and founder of the Mayo Clinic. See www.veirons.com/naturallaw.htm.

Smoking

If you are not a smoker, you may wish to simply skip ahead to the next section: Alcohol on page 51. The following article is extracted from *The Tao of Detox* by Daniel Reid.

From the point of view of health, the best advice on smoking is this: Do not smoke!

While not every substance that is smoked is addictive, smoking itself is highly habit-forming, and while some smokes may be marginally more harmful than others, the real damage to health is caused by smoking itself, not by the particular substance smoked. Smoking involves the inhalation of highly toxic byproducts of combustion, many of which are carcinogenic. 'Where there is smoke there is fire', and when fire burns dried plant material such as tobacco, not only does it produce searing hot smoke, it also produces extremely poisonous chemicals that damage the delicate lining of the bronchia and lungs, cause highly acid forming reactions in the blood and leave harmful toxic residues in the tissues. So unless you have more than recreational reasons for smoking, it is simply not worth the risk.

Nevertheless, all kinds of people throughout the world choose to smoke and, like everything else in life, there are relatively good ways and bad ways to conduct a smoking habit, especially for those who smoke primarily as a means of balancing the nervous system and stimulating cerebral functions. During the 1950s, the renowned clairvoyant healer Edgar Cayce sometimes advised clients to smoke 3-8 cigarettes of tobacco per day to control the symptoms of nervous disorders and compensate for inherent imbalances in their neurochemistry. It did not matter whether the client already smoked or not, but Cayce stipulated that in order to gain the desired therapeutic effects without harming health, it was essential not to exceed his recommended daily dosage of 3-8 cigarettes.

Tobacco is a potent medicinal herb with strong natural affinity for brain and nerve tissues. Even in very moderate doses such as those recommended by Cayce, tobacco stimulates abundant secretions of a wide range of vital neurotransmitters that are essential for balanced brain functions. In Cayce's time, cigarettes were not yet contaminated with dioxin and the hundreds of other carcinogenic chemicals that are used to manufacture cigarettes today, so they were still a relatively safe product, especially when used according to Cayce's guidelines. For people who cannot think clearly or function properly in society due to nervous disorders caused by inherent or acquired imbalances in their neurochemistry, the moderate risks to health posed by smoking 3-8 cigarettes made with pure tobacco and rolled in chemical-free paper are certainly acceptable, if that is what it takes to control their symptoms. As long as smokers do not exceed such a moderate daily dosage, they can gain significant therapeutic benefits from smoking tobacco, at minimum cost to health, and the smoking habit can become more helpful than harmful.

Similarly, many people today suffering from the advanced stages of cancer and AIDS report that smoking a bit of cannabis hemp stimulates their appetites and restores their capacity to digest food and assimilate nutrition, while also relieving the intense physical pain caused by their conditions and allowing them to sleep soundly at night.

Prior to its prohibition, opium was also smoked as much for its medicinal benefits as for pleasure. In fact, during the 18th and 19th centuries in China, traditional doctors often recommended that elderly people suffering from chronic pain and incurable degenerative conditions associated with ageing start smoking opium in moderate daily dosages in order to control their discomfort and permit them to continue enjoying life. While certainly addictive, opium is no more so than tobacco, and smoking opium is considerably less harmful to health than smoking either tobacco or hemp, as evidenced by the remarkable longevity of many old Chinese opium smokers who properly conducted their habits and never exceeded their daily measure.

Today, however, both opium and hemp are prohibited, and tobacco is the only neuro-active medicinal herb that may be smoked legally for recreational or therapeutic purposes. Smokers should be aware, however, that tobacco is at least as addictive as opium, and that it is an even more difficult addiction to break than opiates; smoking tobacco is also more hazardous to health than smoking either hemp or opium. Nevertheless, since tobacco remains the only legal and socially condoned form of smoking throughout most of the world today, we shall limit our discussion here to tobacco.

Cigarettes

If you smoke cigarettes, the best advice is not to exceed Edgar Cayce's recommended daily allowance of 3-8 cigarettes, and to strictly follow this cardinal rule: Roll your own, or leave them alone. Factory-made cigarettes today truly live up to their designation as 'coffin nails', but what causes lung cancer and eventually kills the smoker is not the tobacco - it is the carcinogenic chemicals added to the tobacco and the paper in the cigarette production process.

Among the approximately 2,000 toxic chemicals commonly found in commercially produced cigarettes today, dioxin poses the greatest threat to human health. Dioxin is a proven carcinogen that not only causes cancer but also produces genetic mutations, reproductive defects and brain damage. According to the Environmental Protection Agency in America, 'dioxin is by far the most toxic chemical known to mankind', and a report issued by a group of distinguished German scientists in 1998 concludes that dioxin alone is responsible for at least 12 per cent of all human cancers in industrialized societies. A UK study published in 1998 made it clear that dioxin can cause breast cancer in rats. The researchers exposed pregnant rats to small amounts of dioxin on the 15th day of pregnancy; the female offspring of the dioxin-exposed rats were born normal, but by the time they were seven weeks old, their mammary glands had developed an unusually high number of 'terminal end buds' - the places in the breast where cancers develop. This is definitely not something you want to inhale from the burning tip of a cigarette - not unless you are trying to kill yourself.

Many popular brands of cigarette today also contain radioactive residues from the uranium dust which commercial growers add to the chemical fertilizers they use on their tobacco crops. Why on earth they add radioactive material to the soil in which tobacco is grown has not been explained, but traces of radioactive isotopes of uranium are present in their products as well as in the lungs of people who smoke them. No wonder the Marlboro Man succumbed to lung cancer at the height of his fame.

The paper used to manufacture ready-made cigarettes is even more contaminated with poisonous chemicals than the tobacco itself. Cigarette smokers who are still reluctant to take the time to roll their own cigarettes should try this experiment: cut open a typical popular brand of cigarette, remove the tobacco, flatten out the paper, and lay it in an ashtray; with the glowing tip of a lit cigarette, touch one corner of the paper and observe what happens. The edge of the paper ignites and the entire sheet gradually incinerates to ash, without bursting into flame, with the glowing edge fizzling and sparkling like the fuse of a firecracker as it eats its way through the paper until it is gone. The chemicals added to cigarette paper to produce this effect are similar to those used in making fuses for firecrackers and other explosives, and the reason they're added is to make sure that the cigarette continues burning even when the smoker isn't puffing on it, in order to increase consumption and sales of cigarettes.

Smokers accustomed to the convenience of ready-made factory cigarettes may find rolling their own a chore at first, but it is not nearly as inconvenient as getting lung cancer. Here again, if health and longevity are important considerations, the 'cost/ benefit' ratio of smoking 'coffin nails' compared with that of rolling your own cigarettes clearly dictates that you roll your own.

Good quality, organically grown tobaccos that are free of chemical additives and radioactive residues are now available on the market, and while they may be somewhat more expensive than commercial factory brands, if you roll your own cigarettes and smoke moderately, your consumption will decline so much that it offsets the extra cost of buying pure tobacco. It is equally important to use pure cigarette papers that have not been chemically treated to make them burn faster, and these too are readily available in tobacco shops. One of the purest cigarette papers is Club brand, made by S. D. Modiano of Italy. These have no gum or glue and are thin as a butterfly's wing, yielding a minimum of toxic wastes when burned.[12]

~~~

For an interesting article entitled *Smoking Helps Protect Against Lung Cancer*, see the Joe Vialls Article online[13]. Quote: "This is clue number-one in unraveling the absurd but entrenched Western medical lie that 'smoking causes lung cancer.'"

Alcohol

If you do not drink more than 1 unit of alcohol per day (1 glass of wine or 1 tot of spirits or 1 beer, you may wish to simply skip ahead to the next section: Extending One's Healthy Lifespan to 120 or More on page 55. The following article is extracted from *The Tao of Detox* by Daniel Reid.

'Fire water' is the term which native American tribes used to describe the rum and other liquors brought to North America by British and European colonists. Alcohol intoxication contributed heavily to the downfall of traditional tribal cultures in North America, just as it did in Australia when British settlers introduced 'devil rum' to the indigenous aboriginal tribes there. The blood, liver and brain chemistry of these genetic groups are unable to properly metabolize alcohol, resulting in devastating destructive effects on their bodies and minds whenever it is consumed. For this reason, alcohol still remains a 'forbidden fruit' in many traditional tribal cultures, as well as in most Islamic countries and many parts of India, where its consumption is strictly prohibited and severely punished.

In the Western world, however, from early Greek and Roman times to the present day, alcohol has always been the main intoxicant of choice, and liquor is consumed in more variety and volume than anywhere else on earth. When Westerners began to colonize parts of Asia during the 17th and 18th centuries, they brought their liquor and drinking habits with them, prompting native observers to remark, 'Liquor is to the white man as mother's milk is to babies'.

From the viewpoint of traditional Eastern medicine, 'fire water' is actually a very apt term for alcohol. When alcohol is metabolized, it produces a lot of heat in the body, and if consumed daily in large amounts, this constant metabolic 'fire' tends to 'burn out' the internal

---

[12] *The Tao of Detox* by Daniel Reid, Simon & Schuster, 2003
[13] www.vialls.com/transpositions/smoking.html

organs, particularly the liver and brain. Alcohol is also a potent solvent of organic matter, which means it can dissolve organic tissue such as brain and liver cells, and its metabolism in the body is extremely acid-forming. As previously noted, high acidity is also regarded as a condition of yang excess, so drinking 'fire water' produces extremely yang conditions of 'fire-energy excess' both as excess heat and excess acidity.

The first drink or two of any liquor has a swift stimulating effect on human metabolism, producing a fast flush of body heat and a big surge of extra physical and mental energy. However, if the drinker continues to drink, the excess acidity and toxic waste produced in the blood and tissues by the continuous metabolism of alcohol accumulate rapidly, overloading the system with toxic metabolites and rapidly depleting reserves of vital nutrients and energy. As the body struggles to process and excrete the toxins and quell the metabolic 'fire' more alcohol enters the bloodstream with each sip, adding more fuel to the fire and progressively weakening the body's vital functions.

At the same time, the intoxication produced in the mind as a side effect of the toxic influence of alcohol on brain and nerve tissues continues to grow more intense with each drink, disorienting the drinker's mind and producing a drunken stupor that ends in loss of consciousness. The toxic metabolite of alcohol which causes the most damage to brain and nerve cells, and which destroys liver tissue, is acetaldehyde. This highly reactive, extremely toxic acid poisons the bloodstream and corrodes the cells and tissues. Crude cheap liquor, which produces far more of this toxic acid waste in the body than more refined forms of alcohol, is known among derelict drinkers as 'rot-gut' because of the highly corrosive effects of this compound on the internal organs.

Contrary to popular notions, the forms of alcohol that are most hazardous to human health are not 'hard' liquors such as whisky and rum but rather the fermented varieties such as beer and wine. Although beer and wine have a lower percentage of alcohol than distilled spirits, fermented liquors retain all of the metabolic wastes produced by the yeast during the fermentation process - in effect 'yeast poop' - and these fermentive wastes are highly acid-forming and toxic to the tissues. The liver bears the major burden of processing all the acids and toxic wastes that enter the body and pollute the bloodstream whenever beer and wine are drunk and, if fermented liquors are consumed daily, the liver gradually succumbs to toxic overload, swelling up and hardening with residual toxic waste until cirrhosis develops.

To make matters worse, most commercial beers and wines today contain chemical contaminants such as formaldehyde, preservatives, artificial dyes, flavoring agents and other toxic additives, all of which contribute more to blood acidosis, tissue toxicity and the gradual erosion of the liver. In terms of their effects on health and longevity, except for an occasional glass of an exceptionally good vintage or brew with dinner, beer and wine are not good choices as intoxicants for daily use, especially for 'social drinking', when one tends to drink to excess, because the 'cost/benefit' ratio is far too high.

Distilled spirits, which are refined from fermented liquors, are a much 'cleaner' form of alcohol for human consumption because the distillation process completely eliminates all the other toxic by-products of fermentation, leaving only pure distilled alcohol. While distilled spirits such as vodka and brandy have a higher alcohol content than beer or wine, they are usually consumed in much smaller amounts per drink than fermented beverages, and therefore they deliver the same basic dose of alcohol into the bloodstream.

Known for centuries in Western Europe as eau de vie, the 'water of life', and in ancient China as jiou-jing, the 'essence of wine', distilled spirits were originally used more for therapeutic, medicinal purposes than for recreational intoxication. Used properly and in moderation, spirits have potent medicinal properties that may be used to treat a variety of conditions, including sluggish circulation, insufficient body heat, low metabolic rate and nervous tension. The slightly intoxicating effect on the mind produced by small doses of spirits adds an extra dimension to its therapeutic applications, and this psycho-active influence is well reflected in the term chosen to denote distilled alcohol - spirits.

All distilled spirits, including brandy and whisky, are crystal clear and completely pure after the distillation process. The distinctive amber color and characteristic flavor in various types of whisky, brandy and other tinted spirits come from the resins leached from the wooden casks in which these liquors are aged. This aging process leaves tannins and other toxic resins suspended in the spirits, and these must all be processed by the liver along with the toxic metabolites of alcohol itself. Therefore, the healthiest choice in spirits are the clear varieties that have not been aged in wooden casks, such as vodka, gin, tequila and white rum.

Throughout East Asia, people drink a type of medicinal spirit prepared by steeping potent tonic herbs in distilled spirits for three to six months, then straining the infused liquor into bottles and taking it in measured dosages on a daily basis, particularly in the winter. Known in China as yao jiou ('medicine liquor') or chwun-jiou ('spring wine'), this ancient herbal tonic has been used for thousands of years throughout the Far East as a means of preserving health, boosting vitality and prolonging life, as well as for its relaxing effects. The alcohol extracts and preserves all the essential active ingredients from the various tonic herbs, delivering them swiftly into the bloodstream directly through the stomach and providing a strong metabolic boost to the therapeutic potency of the herbal essences. Medicinal spirits are an excellent delivery system for the life-prolonging therapeutic benefits of herbal tonics such as ginseng, astragalus and wolfberry, while also serving the 'recreational' function of liquor. This is a good example of how the 'art of rational retox' may be applied to transform a 'toxic intoxicant' into a 'tonic intoxicant', thereby reducing the costs to health and increasing the benefits to longevity of drinking alcohol.[14]

Tips for Tipplers & Smokers

If you drink and/or smoke daily, it is important to take a few basic precautions to counteract the additional acidity, toxicity and dehydration which alcohol and tobacco produce in the body. Alcohol in particular dehydrates the blood and tissues, and it is therefore necessary to drink a few extra glasses of alkaline water each day, both to flush out the toxic acid wastes and to re-hydrate the blood and cellular fluids. If the water you drink is charged with negative ions, it has even greater detoxifying and re-hydrating activity in the tissues and helps protect the liver from damage by the toxic metabolites of alcohol and tobacco in the bloodstream.

People who smoke and drink regularly should also take extra rations of antioxidant nutrients, particularly vitamins E, C and beta carotene, plus a full spectrum mineral supplement to replace the essential minerals and trace elements depleted from the tissues by alcohol and tobacco. It is also a good idea to take some form of 'green food' supplement as a source of organic chlorophyll and other cleansing elements to purify the blood and cellular fluids.

One of the most effective antidotes of all against the toxic damage caused by daily use of alcohol, tobacco and other intoxicants is to drink High Mountain Oolung Tea (gao-shan oolung cha), especially first thing in the morning and again late in the afternoon, which is how many smokers and drinkers in China, Taiwan and Japan protect their bodies from the hazards of their habits. Recent scientific research has confirmed the efficacy of High Mountain Oolung Tea as a potent blood purifier, tissue detoxificant, alkalizer and preventive against cancer. It is particularly effective in preventing toxic damage to the tissues of the lungs and the liver, which are precisely the organs that smokers and drinkers must take special measures to purify and protect. Here again we see how the 'art of rational retox' transforms an ordinary daily

---

[14] *The Tao of Detox* by Daniel Reid, Simon & Schuster, 2003

beverage such as tea into an extraordinary therapeutic drink that protects health and prolongs life.[15]

Extending One's Healthy Lifespan to 120 or More

Earlier we mentioned that one of the Immutable Laws of Nature is that of easily living to 120, not the commonly held belief of 70 or 80 years. Here we discuss how achieving such longevity is possible.

A Suppressed Longevity Therapy

There is a much suppressed breakthrough therapy involving Free Radical Pathology and Bio Oxidative Medicine, that involves the single greatest event in medical history. This therapy affects all forms of life-shortening diseases from AIDS to cancer, the common cold to flu, arthritis to asthma, Alzheimer's to atherosclerosis. It is also used to improve performance of Olympic athletes and race horses. Even if you are not ill, it could increase energy, give clearer thinking and make you feel a lot better; making living to 120 a reasonable goal.. This therapy is known for indefinitely extended 'middlescence'.

Why has it been withheld? Why has this proven 'miracle' treatment been assigned 'fraud' status? Welcome to the real world. When things do not make sense, check out the money trail.

Too many health professionals have too much to lose. Anesthetists, operating team personnel, coronary care unit staff, radiologists, technicians, hospital administrators - some forty-five specialists in all - stand to have their years of training and sizeable pay checks wiped out. Self-serving proponents continue to withhold facts, misrepresent and distort benefits and viciously oppose the one therapy that might doom them to the unemployment lines.

That is without the influence of the behind-the-scenes shenanigans of pharmaceutical, medical and food industry cronies. The average citizen would be shocked to know of the extent to which these powerhouses are able to distort science news, as we have already discussed.

On 4 April 1991 Kay Pierson, a Washington DC anti-trust lawyer presented the FTC (Federal Trade Commission) with a 75-page fact-filled document supporting her allegation that the parties charged are involved in a conspiracy to stop the growth and development of alternative medicine.

The Health Insurance Industry just cannot afford to have this therapy approved. Why? It would be too costly. Because not just the currently ill, but anyone over 21 (and many kids) probably can establish a valid basis for needing and demanding this therapy, due to

---

[15] *The Tao of Detox* by Daniel Reid, Simon & Schuster, 2003

the damage being done to us by environmental factors about which authorities are equally loath to inform us. The treatment of which we speak is Chelation Therapy.

What Can This Therapy Do?

A case could be made that it is easier to name an ailment that it does not correct than to list those conditions it is known to relieve. Unanticipated benefits in place of toxic side-effects from drugs reverses or reduces:

- senility,
- schizophrenia,
- rheumatoid arthritis,
- osteoarthritis,
- gout,
- kidney stones,
- stroke-related coma,
- gall bladder stones,
- multiple sclerosis,
- lupus,
- Parkinson's Disease,
- Lou Gherig's Disease,
- osteoporosis,
- hypertension,
- memory loss,
- scleroderma,
- Raynaud's Disease,
- digitalis intoxication,
- intermittent claudication,
- emphysema,
- diabetic ulcers,
- leg ulcers,
- venomous snake bite,
- impotence,
- emotional difficulties,
- high insulin levels,
- high blood cholesterol,
- high blood pressure,
- normalization of cardiac arrhythmias,
- leg muscle cramps,
- allergies,
- weight control,
- heart contractions,
- varicose veins,
- age spots,
- aches and pains,
- hair loss,
- diuretics,
- cold extremities,
- chronic fatigue,
- memory and concentration,
- post cataract vision,
- vision and hearing problems and many other signs of aging.

Table 1 – Chelation Therapy Cures

As you can see, there is very little that this radical new therapy cannot cure, and yet it is purposely suppressed, because of the risk of reduced profits for the greedy medical community.

We discuss Chelation Therapy in more detail in Chapter 14.

9. Independent Wealth Creation

Attaining the proper reasoning skills and the base of knowledge to manage private profits and build strategic wealth requires attention to a 4-Step Foundational Wealth-Building Process:

- **Learning**: Acquiring knowledge and information
- **Unlearning**: Discarding and shedding false understanding and assumptions
- **Relearning**: Absorbing truth-filled insights
- **Living**: Adjusting life purposes and interactions to reflect added knowledge and understanding.

Before diving into the essence of Independent Wealth Creation, it is important that we again remind you of the following points:

- At no point will you be working for, on behalf of, or for the benefit of Freedom Technology.
- We are not some sort of Multi Level Marketing (MLM) organization.
- You will be keeping everything you make as a result of implementing these strategies.
- You agree that you are solely responsible for seeking the necessary professional advice before implementing any of the strategies we are going to teach.

Some have asked why we accept no responsibility for your business venture. Well, since you are not sharing the profits with us, you cannot expect us to carry the can if you mess it up. All we are doing is giving you our very best advice and knowledge, gained over years and years of running successful, money-making businesses. You are fully and totally responsible for your success or failure in applying these concepts and strategies.

Right, let us get started.

What is Independent Wealth Creation?

Let us get one thing straight first. There is absolutely no magic road to riches. If you have been conned out of your hard-earned money before by some slick sales person telling you he will turn you into a millionaire overnight, you will know what we mean. It cannot be done.

There are only three ways of accumulating enough money to live a totally free and fulfilled life. They are:

1. Steal it;
2. Inherit it, or be given it;
3. Run your own business.

Route Number 1 is not a particularly attractive route because of the very real possibility of landing in jail, where of course you cannot enjoy the fruits of your efforts.

Route Number 2 is purely luck. It is great if you are fortunate enough to be handed a wedge of cash, but do not count on it.

That only leaves Route Number 3 - running your own business. For the normal person, who does not inherit or receive wealth, there is only one option, and that is to start your own business and make a success of it.

Salaried Positions

What? You thought that maybe you could get rich by working hard for someone else? For a salary?

Forget trying to become wealthy by working for someone else. It cannot be done.

As a reminder, a hopelessly trapped wage-slave does not stand a chance of making any serious money. We would go further and say that most employed people can hardly even pay their way, let alone accumulate money.

Why?

Because the system is designed to ensure their poverty. The entire system of employment works on the principle of bosses paying the absolute rock-bottom minimum wage which they can legally get away with. This is called *market forces* where the sheep scramble over each other to work for less and less money just to ensure that they have a job.

For you, this means that regardless of how skilled you are or how professional you are, unless you are unique, there is always someone waiting in the wings to grab your job at a lower rate. Therefore by definition you are being paid the absolute *minimum* which can possibly be paid to you.

Faced with this one fact alone, one has to be pretty crazy to want to work for someone else, and yet many people do. Perhaps you are just such a person.

The most common reason people give for choosing full-time employment is 'security'.

Let us be serious: How much job-security is there nowadays? Are you confident you will have the same job 3 months from now? In most Western nations stable salaried positions are becoming more and more scarce, no matter what the Unemployment Figures say. Look at the reality around you – the beggars in the street, a steadily decreasing living standard for all.

Another common reason people give is that they do not know what business to start.

Well that is where *Fresh Wisdom* comes in. A little further in this Life Manual we will show you how easy it is to set up your own independent revenue generator. But before we do, let us discuss a little about money.

What is Money?

Time and space do not permit us to go into the full history of the rape of money through the ages. For now, we will assume that you have some inkling of an idea that money today exists merely on paper, or worse, merely as bits and bytes in computers all over the world. Very few currencies are backed by any real measure of value (like gold or silver).

If you would like to read more on the background of the purposeful debasement of money (and we encourage you to do so), read *The Economic Rape of America*, available free online[16]. While the book is US-centric, the same logic can be applied to any currency and nation.

Historically, only gold and silver have passed the test of history. Our founding fathers knew that any divergence from the use of gold and silver would lead to economic problems.

> *"I deny the power of the general government to making paper money, or anything else a legal tender""* -- Thomas Jefferson

> *"The terms 'lawful money' and 'lawful money of the United States' shall be construed to mean gold or silver coin of the United States."* (12 USC 152)

> *"Legal tender is quite different from lawful money. In no U.S. law are Federal Reserve notes declared to be 'lawful money.' Lawful money is that money described in the Coinage Act of 1792 and in Article I, section 10 of the U.S. Constitution: gold and silver... the only money the Supreme Law of the Land allows states to make legal tender."* -- Tupper Saussy, 1980

We have mentioned these quotes just to show you that money in circulation today is in fact illegal. Very few people realize this, and we would encourage you to do your own research on this, because we would like to move on to another paradigm shift.

Before we do, you may wish to remind yourself of our explanation of *Paradigms and Paradigm Shifts*, which we discussed on page 16. This is very important.

---

[16] www.buildfreedom.com/tl/rape1.shtml

Changing Your View of Money

We have established already that paper money is in fact illegal. We also know that paper money is *fiat money*. The term *fiat money* refers to what people are forced by government decree to use as medium of exchange. The Latin word "fiat" means "let it be done." All paper money, including the U.S. dollar, is fiat money, since our governments do not allow us to use any other currency to, for example, pay our taxes. (Try paying your US taxes with Euro's, or your British taxes with South African Rands, or your Canadian taxes with physical gold, or your Australian taxes in silver coinage – you will not get very far).

So, our governments are forcing us to use illegal money. Or taking this one step further, they are forcing us to break the law every time we perform a financial transaction. Of course, no-one is going to throw you in jail simply for producing US dollars to pay for your groceries in a US supermarket, but that is just the point we are trying to make – breaking the law is not always a black-or-white matter. Laws can be twisted, and very often are by governments.

Now, let us take this matter one step further. In doing so, you may well be shocked at what we are suggesting, but keep in mind; we are just asking you to think about money for what it is: bits and bytes in a computer, nothing more, and nothing less.

When is it Acceptable to Steal Money?

Aaah! We thought that might make you sit up and take notice.

We have already proved that by using fiat money, we are being forced to break the law. It would seem then that fiat money is above and beyond the law. If governments can break the law by forcing us to use it, can we as individuals not 'break the law' too, as far as money is concerned? If money is nothing more than bits and bytes in a computer, can we not use that to our advantage to speed the accumulation thereof?

Before reading any further, we must make this one distinction about 'breaking the law'.

Any criminal activity which harms another human being is against the principles of *Fresh Thinkers*, and will never be entertained. But any activity performed against an already corrupt system cannot be deemed as criminal. This is because no individual is being harmed, and the same principles are being applied as those of the corrupt system.

Read the previous paragraph again before continuing. Notice that we are not promoting anarchy by breaking every law there is (governments should still be respected, even if we do not agree with everything they stand for). The point we are trying to make is that governments break laws every day, and live according to a different set of laws as those imposed on us, their subjects. Which set of laws is correct?

We are getting a bit beyond ourselves here, and are delving into material which we are going to cover much later.

For now, let us just say that, for example, taking a loan from a bank which you have no intention of repaying would ordinarily be considered a crime. However, no individual is harmed, and you are simply moving bits and bytes from the bank's computer into your own account, using their own corrupt system of fiat money.

Morality

We feel it is necessary at this point to take a short time-out to discuss Morality. *Fresh Thinkers* bypass conventional morality. We operate from our own internally generated set of morals which may, or may not agree with the morality of the time and place we find ourselves in.

Read the above sentence again. It has profound implications for you, if you are to gain full advantage of *Fresh Wisdom*.

We take as few decisions as possible because we know that we have hardly any information concerning the actual effect of our decisions.

While others pontificate noisily about 'rights' and 'wrongs', we simply get on with doing something enjoyable and life-enhancing, while understanding the consequences of our actions. We will discuss this in more detail in a future chapter.

Back to the bank loan.

Note that if you were to stop repaying a loan, there would be consequences if you are caught. But if you avoid being caught, this would be a justifiable action taken against an already corrupt system. Incidentally, if this were to happen, you would not end up with a criminal record – simply an adverse credit record. Makes one wonder why there is no criminal record – maybe the banks know that their money system is already illegal and therefore will not press charges? Hmmm…

So to stress, we are not suggesting you take out as many loans as you can with the intention of defaulting. But hopefully this has changed one view you might have about money.

Leverage

The other view of money we need to change is the commonly held view that the amount of money one earns is directly related to the amount of effort expended. You know: if I work overtime this month I will earn enough to go on holiday, or pay all the bills, or whatever.

This is a very limiting belief, and is the one belief mostly responsible for keeping the vast majority of salaried slaves 'average'.

And yet this need not be the case at all. By learning to leverage your time, you can apply creative effort just once and continue to generate revenue from that once-off effort.

The best examples of the concept of leverage are pop stars. Let us use Britney Spears as a specific example. During her early teenage years she worked really hard writing and singing songs and recording high impact music videos which sold exceptionally well. After a number of years of hard work and tremendous success, she married, stopped recording and got fat. Of course, she can afford to not have to work for a very long time, because her ongoing album sales are still earning her a significant royalty, even though she is no longer performing. She did the work once, up front, and now continues to reap the rewards. That is leverage, and it is a very powerful concept.

Now that we have shattered two major myths we have about money, let us see if we can apply any of our newly discovered principles into a new Independent Wealth Creation Machine.

Dot Com's Are Not Dead!

If you have never thought of running your own business, or are already running a small business and struggling, then here is a little golden nugget of advice:

Drop everything you are doing right now and take a good, long, hard look at selling a product on the Internet.

If you are in the online marketing business already, then please be patient. In subsequent chapters we will be giving you some incredible information which could increase your conversion rate by up to one hundred times. But there are some reading this who have never considered using the Internet for anything other than surfing and browsing, so we have a little educating to do.

The real world is no place for a small or home-based business. At least not if you want to double or triple your income every year. There is only one place that this type of rapid income growth can perpetuate: in cyberspace. Only online can a tiny-budget business experience rapid growth in income.

There are many reasons for this. Among them are the tiny operating costs, a global customer base, and the ability to continue selling 24 hours a day, even while you sleep.

Here is something worth considering:

Very few corporations and conglomerates ever provide true *value for money*.

How can that be possible? We keep hearing that phrase all the time: *value for money*.

Exactly. It is another way we have been conned into buying things from mega-corporations: by being told we are getting *value for money*. It is seldom found these days. To make a profit, any large business has to sell things for more money than they are really worth. To do this, they merely convince prospects that the goods are worth what they are paying for them. This is the basis of all advertising, and when you buy anything, from a packet of crisps to a BMW, you are paying way, way, way over and above what the product is really worth. Otherwise how could all those middle men possibly make their cuts?

And this is the true beauty of selling an Information Product on the Internet. Information has *perceived* value, and yet costs miniscule amounts to produce and deliver. So an item which costs very little to produce, nothing to store (it is digital, so it is stored in bits and bytes) and peanuts to deliver (it is sent via email instead of by Express Mail), can easily be sold for $20 to $50 apiece. And because you have a global market, hundreds or thousands of these products can be sold monthly.

Are you beginning to understand the beauty of selling Information Products on the Internet?

Phenomenal successes abound on the Internet. In mid-2004, one entrepreneur made more than $1 million in one day![17]

So what do you need to succeed in this business?

You need a helping hand from a team which has been in this game for more than 5 years. And that team is none other than Freedom Technology, publishers of *Fresh Wisdom*. Seriously, we have spent years learning the hard way, and we are applying those lessons learnt by making it easy for you to succeed online too. Believe us, it is a total jungle out there, and without someone to show you the way, you will almost certainly *lose* money at this game. But if you follow our advice, we promise that you will have absolutely the best chance of establishing a leveraged passive income generator, with *minimum* risk.

We are prepared to teach you, if you are prepared to learn. We will tell you every little wrinkle, every little dodge and we will hold absolutely nothing back.

But be warned!

If you have ever looked at online money making strategies before, you will already know what to prepare yourself for. If you have never considered this lucrative form of leveraging your time to earn money even while you sleep, let us warn you now that by blindly going online and starting your search, you will be bombarded by erroneous, distorted, inaccurate, puffed up, and overpriced advice and strategies about how to make money online.

---

[17] www.milliondollarday.com/

Here is another harsh truth: 99% of the information you will be swamped with is rehashed by so-called Internet Marketing Guru's (self-proclaimed, by the way). Practically every single one of the products that will be offered has its origins in the works of the following people (in no particular order):

Claude Hopkins,
Emanuel Haldeman-Julius,
Raymond Rubicam,
Maxwell Sackheim,
James Webb Young,
Rosser Reeves,
David Ogilvy,
Alvin Eicoff,
J Douglass Edwards,
Jay Abraham,
Gary Halbert,
Leo Burnett, and
George Cecil.

The pathway to true Internet wealth has become blurred because of garbage marketing information, dished out by Internet wannabes, that railroads everyone who uses it.

To make matters worse, for every success on the Internet there are at least 10,000 failures, possibly far more (no accurate study has ever been conducted). Let us get down to the truth: at least 98% of all the individuals who start marketing on the Internet will not make a single solitary dime.

Why the High Failure Rate?

Because they either do not have the right product or they cannot connect with buyers for their product. It is as simple as that.

So if the failure rate is so high and it is so difficult to find reliable information, you may be asking yourself why on earth we are recommending that you consider selling a product on the Internet?

Because, once you have the discipline to ignore the hundreds of slick sales letters you will come across online and understand the principles we are about to share with you, it really is easy to make money online.

Now listen carefully, because you will not find this information summarized as succinctly anywhere. Get this right and you will be able to break free from the bondage of a salaried job, forever.

Seven Power Steps to Making Money on the Internet

Power Step 1: Own a web site that sells products using the direct response principle. In other words have a hard-hitting, direct sales letter on your site, with no other confusing links and offers. Your sales letter should follow the AIDA principle:

- It must attract *Attention*,
- It must continually draw *Interest* as the prospect is reading it,
- It must create *Desire* and finally,
- It must demand *Action* now.

(We will show you how to do this.)

Power Step 2: Sell what the public wants and will pay money for. It is the law of Supply and Demand. In other words, do not try to sell something that only you have a passion for. (We will show you how to find what people are searching for online.)

Power Step 3: Own your product 100%. In other words, do not sell affiliate products as your primary source of income. (We will show you how easy it is to create your own digital information products which can be downloaded instantly from the Internet once you have received payment.)

Power Step 4: Control the price of what you sell online, and constantly test which price, which ad copy, which bonus, and which guarantee offers the greatest return. In other words, never stop testing and tweaking your sales letter. (We will show you how easy it is to test two versions of an advert simultaneously.)

Power Step 5: Own a private list of subscribers who have asked you to keep in contact with them. Build trust and a relationship with them by regularly sending them brief, fresh, useful information that can change their lives.

Power Step 6: Set up to instantly accept credit card orders online. If you are going to make money you have to be able to take payments made directly to you - not to a third party who may or may not pay you at some point in the future.

Power Step 7: Promote your products like crazy, or you will not be making any sales whatsoever. Forget what the experts say about getting free traffic to your brand new website - their techniques are outdated in the constantly changing world of online marketing. (We will show you the most effective promotion tactics which, although not free, give excellent return on your investment.)

Some of these steps may be a little confusing right now, because we are throwing a lot of new information on the table. But in the next chapter of Independent Wealth Creation we are going to show you exactly what we mean. We cannot get ahead of ourselves just yet.

The Internet Wealth Creation Secret

We are often asked: "What is the secret of how the 'Big Names' make their money online?"

Well, we are not going to make any friends, but here is the truth: *There is no secret.* No matter what various courses or books tell you, no matter how many gurus shout it from the rooftops that they have the only secret to making money online, there is no magic formula.

We are shooting ourselves in the foot here. We hope you appreciate this, so listen up.

You will only ever get rich working for yourself. If you are part of an MLM, or selling someone else's affiliate product, then you are not working for yourself. Sure, you can make a comfortable income selling or in an MLM, but you will never become wealthy and there is always someone above you making more.

You bought this book because, among other reasons, you want to become independently wealthy. To do that, you must get other people to give you money.

All straightforward so far?

If there really is a secret to making money online, here it is (and you will not find this anywhere else):

Listen to what the experts say, copy their techniques, but do not fall for their convincing.

Buying yet another book, course, tape or DVD series or attending a seminar will not make you a millionaire.

These 'experts' are good at what they do. They are good at convincing you to part with your hard earned cash. They will convince you that they are your personal friends and they will make you believe that they will make you millions.

You are after a short cut. You are after a quick buck. So... you are susceptible to these promises.

They have thousands of affiliates selling their products, signing people up and promoting like crazy. Each affiliate is hoping to get rich by earning 30-50% on whatever they are selling. Some make it, most do not, but the winners are always the people at the top.

So how do you become wealthy?
-   Copy these experts;
-   Create or obtain your own product;
-   Get other people selling for you.

Everything we have told you not to accept for yourself, do to others. This is difficult for some people to do, but we are telling you the truth.

It is your task to get others to believe in you. It is your task to take their money. Build your own service, write your own eBook or develop your own product. Then sell it. That is the only way to become wealthy.

If you latch on to every word the experts say, you will get caught in the trap of spending, spending and more spending. You will be buying eBooks, buying tapes, attending seminars, buying expensive domains, websites and mailing servers.

You do not need any of this.

But we are getting way ahead of ourselves. The purpose of today's lesson was purely to introduce you to the idea of selling a product on the Internet, and warn you that there are slick salesmen out there trying to extricate as much cash from you as possible. Beware of them.

One final word, in case you have not fully understood what we are trying to say: There is only one low-risk, legal way of creating a leveraged, passive income stream. This way is to start your own online business. And it is fun, too. Most normal businesses are a first class pain in the rear-end. They require lots of money at the start. They require your life's efforts for at least five years before the rewards start flowing in. Most normal businesses fail within two years of start-up, resulting in huge personal losses for the owners. We say, "Forget all that". We suggest starting a business which requires no premises, no staff, no overheads (to speak of), and most importantly - no large start-up capital. We will be telling you exactly how to start this business from scratch, the cheapskate's way. When you start making profit from your business, then you can spend a little on improving the business - but not before.

And we are very excited to tell you about a marketing vehicle we have created just for you. We will do all the advertising for your newly created product, and you keep all the revenue. But this is way, way ahead of where we are at now. We will tell you about these details towards the end of the book. We just had to mention it now, because it is so exciting we are just busting to tell you. But all in due course...

Debt

Now we want to hit you hard with a statement which might surprise you, because it comes from a lesson which we have not yet covered. It has to do with making you wealthy. It has to do with money, and it is worth mentioning to you now.

It is important to have total control over impulse consumption on credit.

What do we mean?

Very simply, ensuring that your debt is well-managed, and always within control. *Fresh Thinkers* understand the workings of debt, and understand that well managed debt enhances liquidity and therefore freedom of action.

But one of the main secrets of becoming wealthy is first to control debt. It took us ages and ages to learn this simply stated fact. Wealthy people kept telling us this 'secret' but we refused to listen. In fact we thought you had to borrow lots of money to become rich. You know, to 'invest' in your company, to make it grow, etc. Well we were wrong. There are numerous examples of small businesses that have lost everything because a bank walked in and shut the operations down when debt was not serviced properly. We will be returning to this subject again in a later section, but we wanted to warn you about it early on.

The other reason we mention it now, is because selling a product online is the only legitimate business we know of that you can start without going into serious debt.

~~~

Never forget that the purpose for which a man lives is the improvement of the man himself, so that he may go out of this world having, in his great sphere or his small one, done some little good for his fellow creatures and labored a little to diminish the sin and sorrow that are in the world. – W.E. Gladstone

We are here on earth to do good for others. What the others are here for, I don't know. – W.H. Auden

A useless life is an early death. - Goethe

No nation ancient or modern ever lost the liberty of freely speaking, writing, or publishing their sentiments, but forthwith lost their liberty in general and became slaves. – John P. Zenger

There is a wonderful mythical law of nature that the three things we crave most in life -- happiness, freedom, and peace of mind -- are always attained by giving them to someone else. - Peyton Conway March

10. Spiritual and Metaphysical Truths

We will be discussing religion in this chapter, and for many this is an extremely contentious topic, so it is important to lay a few foundations first. If you are currently fairly open-minded about religion, or follow no particular religion, you may wish to skip ahead to How Religion Affects Our World View on page 70.

But if you currently hold extremely deep-rooted religious beliefs, or avidly follow a particular religion, no matter what it is, please take the time to read these introductory paragraphs.

Religion is a touchy subject – deeply personal and often fiercely defended. It is also the one area where many are more deeply enslaved than any other area.

So far we have covered 3 of the 5 Essential Pillars of Fulfilled Living. Our guess is that you have learned a few new things, but nothing that has been said so far was impossible to believe, given a little thoughtful analysis.

Oh how we wish the same were true for religion, the penultimate and possibly most important of the Essential Pillars of Fulfilled Living. (In the next chapter we will be covering Individual Sovereignty and True Freedom. We cannot progress to this level until we have covered Religion).

For this section, we must ask you simply to keep an open mind (or rather a rational, active mind), since we are not attacking any specific religion, yours included. We have mentioned before that some illusions would seem obvious to you - hardly worth stating, while other illusions you would find almost unbearable to be parted from. Well, if you are religious, then this section will be tough going for you.

It might help if you remember that for many readers, the 'shocking truth' about religion will seem laughably obvious - hardly worth mentioning. At the same time you may get hot under the collar and want to challenge everything that is covered in this section. Remember, all we are trying to do is break free from belief systems which might be illusions. Religion often falls into this category.

We hope you will be open-minded enough to hear us out on this critical pillar of Fulfilled Living. As we said in the introduction: we have to tell you the blunt truth. Some find the material you are about to read shocking or even offensive. In short, they do not like having their security blanket snatched away from them. But power, vitality and a fulfilled life are obtained only by waking up to the truth about yourself and the world.

Are you prepared to stick with us and listen for the ring of truth?

How Religion Affects Our World View

This, the Metaphysical aspect of the 5 Pillars of Fulfilled Living, is the foundation of *Fresh Wisdom*. Here we establish ultimate reality and truth. Until we have achieved this, we do not have a basis for building a life which is truly fulfilling and free.

This implies a process, or following a chain (like the DNA strand). If this chain is correct and accurate, then a true foundation of life can be established.

What we are building through this manual is a way of life, a path that leads to enlightenment and fulfillment, heart-peace, satisfaction and joy. A life lived to the full, where you are truly alive and vibrant, becoming all you were meant to be, recognizing the powers within and exercising them fully, and discovering your true purpose in life.

To achieve the fulfilled life is no simple task. Its accomplishment promises rewards thought by many to be completely unattainable. The cynic has come to doubt that life holds any more than fleeting glimpses of genuine happiness and fulfillment. The one who achieves a reasonable measure of that fulfillment knows that the rewards promised are as genuine as any can be.

Life exacts a toll for rewards.

There is no shortcut to success or happiness.

Violation of eternal principles invariably brings frustration and disappointment. When we determine to comply with eternal truth, fulfillment is the predictable result.

It is our aim and hope that you will be empowered to achieve a wider view of life than the average, leading to true happiness and a fulfilled life.

What is Your World View?

The problems man faces today (social, political, racial, ecological) are a direct result of human behavior.

Human behavior is a dynamic outworking of a world view. If your world view, your life-philosophy, justifies pollution, you will pollute. If it justifies racism, you will be a racist. If it justifies murder, you will have no hesitation in murdering others. If your world view is molded and formed by others who do not have your best interests at heart, you will live an unfulfilled life.

Humanity's problems, behavior, world view and origins are intimately related.

Therefore, resolution of problems depends on a change to proper behavior which demands a change to a correct world view. The point we are trying to make is that the problems of today's (particularly

Western) society cannot be solved without addressing humanity's world view.

As we have stated before, the vast majority have no understanding of a world view, and would be even less inclined to adapt their behavior to one that does not violate the Laws of Nature. So we stress again, that changing everyone's world view, or trying to get the sheep to understand, is an impossible task. It would be easier to move Mount Everest one foot to the left than change society's world view.

And this is why readers of *Fresh Wisdom* comprise a unique group of individuals. We realize that our behavior needs to adapt to achieve a fulfilled life. But at the same time, we realize that we exist within a society which does not and cannot understand our approach to life.

So, no matter what those around us believe and try to impose on us, we understand that:

- A correct world view affects our approach to life which in turn leads to true solutions and a fulfilled life.

To put this another way:

The behavior of each and every society depends on their world view, and the measure of how fulfilled each society is depends very much on their behavior. The two are inextricably linked.

What is My Society's World View?

The obvious question then is "How do I determine whether the society within which I live has a correct world view?"

The best way to determine any value judgment about the specific view held by any society would be to ascertain the results that world view leads to. Analyze these results and then arrive at a conclusion as to whether the specific view relates accurately to truth, which leads to a fulfilled life.

To be specific: Does the society in which I live empower me to live a truly fulfilled life by encouraging a form of behavior which does not violate the Unchanging Laws of Nature?

When asked like this, it would seem obvious to any thinking individual that the typical Western lifestyle and society must be doing something wrong, since few could argue that the society within which we live today offers any teachings or direction on Fulfilled Living.

To go back to our question: Does the society in which I live empower me to live a truly fulfilled life?

Without needing to know the specifics of your culture and your society, *Freedom Technology's* answer is a resounding NO. The authors of *Fresh Wisdom* have lived in many different countries, on all seven continents, enjoying a variety of cultures. Not once have we ever come across a society which empowers its people to live a truly fulfilled life. Some come closer than others, but very few actively encourage fulfilled living.

And many of society's core beliefs have their birth in religion, hence this discussion. Most modern-day religions are man-made and have warped the ideals of Absolute Truth, with the intention of keeping their society enslaved and entrapped. In short, society wants to do everything it can to prevent fulfilled living, and religion is one of the most effective weapons in the battle for control of your mind.

The Con of Religion

Let us dive straight in with another contentious statement:

Religions and cults are man-made inventions designed to allow an elitist priesthood to con value out of those that follow them.

We know that this will upset some, so let us first clear up a few definitions.

Spirituality

Whether gained through life experience, revelation (religious or otherwise) or self-discovery, spirituality is transcendental in nature (meaning beyond the realm and reach of the five senses).

It involves insight and a sense of connection within the self, to others, nature, the Universe or a higher power.

Religion

Religion, in the sense used throughout this manual, is an organized set of beliefs and a way of understanding the Universe and yourself as part of the Universe.

Religion defines (some more strictly than others) how a person's beliefs are expressed and often acts as a guide in terms of how a person expresses his or her spirituality. It aims to provide guidance, perspective, community and support for the individual in his or her solitary practice. By its very definition, religion influences an individual's beliefs.

Throughout this manual we will be discussing religion as defined as an *organized set of beliefs*. We are specifically excluding spirituality from this discussion.

Throughout this manual, the point of reference will be Christianity in all of its many forms. This religion has been singled out purely because it is likely to be the one with which the reader is most familiar. This is the only reason.

However, the comments in this section apply to the vast majority of religions and cults, and any one could have been selected as a point of reference. It is not our intention to embark upon a long and tedious comparison of various religions, because to us, they are all essentially the same; that is, systems designed by one group of people to extract life values from other people. They have little or nothing whatsoever to do with God, or whoever you choose to worship.

We have used the word 'church' to mean any building where any religious ceremonies take place. We have used the word 'God' to mean any Supreme Being, by whatever name you prefer to refer to him or her. We have used the word 'priest' to refer to any religious leader, from any denomination. These terms have purely been chosen for simplicity and ease of reference – no other reason.

So, what is 'religion', understood from the *Fresh Wisdom* point of view?

A religion is a system invented by an elite priesthood who desire to extricate value from their followers.

The priests claim that their mandate comes from a dead, discarnate or supernatural being, and that they are the chosen channels for this power. Having gathered together a flock, the priests then proceed to con values out of the flock under false pretences. In the past, the values were money (in vast quantities) and power.

Although this is still true, more often the values today are respect, kudos, loyalty and power. The priests also enjoy a smug sense of 'doing good'.

Fresh Thinkers choose to see all this for what it is, and quite simply refuse to play. One cannot be religious in the typical sense of the word, and still have power over your own life. The two are completely incompatible.

Religion and Sacrifice

Religion comes in many disguises, but all have a common thread. The message varies from cult to cult, but it is basically a message of sacrifice. Sacrifice your life's pleasures now, so that you might enjoy everlasting life, dwelling with the angels, sitting next to God for all eternity. The words and language might vary, but the message is basically the same.

Throughout history, serious crimes against the people have been committed using the illusion of religion.[18] Millions upon millions of people have been forced to live drab, boring, unfulfilled and painful lives because they have been stifled by religious guilt and fear. It is still going on today. Religion is the single biggest force for evil at large in the world. It causes untold misery and anguish.

Like most of the best illusions, this insidious one exploits several basically good human emotions, e.g. the natural sense of

---

[18] www.infidels.org/library/modern/james_haught/holy.html

wonder, awe and amazement which any thinking person cannot help but feel when confronted with the great, mysterious Universe. Most thinking people have a deep (if uncultivated) sense of mystery, and cannot help but question their place in the cosmic scheme of things. It is to this pure and wonderful human emotion that the cancer of religion attaches itself. It then proceeds to weave a thick web of deceit, lies and illusion which destroys the victim's natural sense of wonder, and replaces it with misery, anguish and hypocrisy.

One cannot become fully empowered and subscribe to any man-made religion. Why?

Because one cannot become a free and enlightened human being and subscribe to a complete fantasy.

If you are religious in any conventional sense, then it will hinder your personal growth until such time as you are strong enough to see through the illusion of religion. If you are religious, then you are extremely likely to dismiss this whole section anyway. However, you will be unable to cross the barrier to personal freedom for as long as you refuse to face up to reality and truth.

We know this is tough. Did you not find it very difficult to accept when you discovered that Santa Claus was not real? That is part of the growing process. Few would disagree that it would be a great handicap to an adult if he were to continue to believe in Santa Claus, the Tooth Fairy and the Easter Bunny. However, the blind following of a man-made religion is a far more dangerous and cancerous fairy-tale.

This is because most people who join religious groups do so because of feelings of fear, guilt and insecurity, and almost never from a position of spontaneous joy of life and desire for knowledge or truth, even though people often delude themselves that they are coming from this position.

This does not mean that we are insensitive to the wonder and mystery of the Universe. We realize that the wonders of the Universe, and the mystery of creation are far greater than the teachings of any man-made religion.

The authors have deliberately avoided the catch-22 of describing our own religious background. This would be a lose-lose scenario. If we told you we were ex-Christians, then you can smile smugly and say: "Ah yes, they obviously had a bad experience, but they do not understand the TRUE message of Jesus". On the other hand, if we tell you that we have never been in a church in our lives, and have zero interest in religion, then you can nod sagely and say: "Ah yes, they do not know what they are talking about due to their lack of experience. I will pray that one day they will discover the love of Christ." Either way, you get a great chance to pigeon-hole us and dismiss the vital message contained in this section. You can then nod-off to sleep again, secure in the knowledge that our message is invalid.

Never forget that religion is an invention of man, not God. Religions are founded by men who claim that God spoke directly to them. They then ask the rest of us to believe it. Furthermore, never forget that religion is a prime illusion used to control the masses by those who seek power - and this means today, now.

Classes of Religious Con Artists

The religious con-artists are not all the same, of course. They seek different levels of power according to their vision. They can be divided into groups as follows (in order of the level of damage they cause to other people's happiness):

1. Evil megalomaniacs who deliberately and calculatingly stir up religious fever and hatred in the masses in order to get them to fight a holy war on their behalf.
2. Power-hungry individuals who divert the masses from thinking about real issues by getting them to expend their energies in religious hatred of another sect. (e.g. Germany 1939, Klu Klux Klan, etc). In these cases, religious hatred is often indistinguishable from race hatred.
3. Clever politicians who exploit religious ill-feeling.
4. Wealthy religious institutions who wish to retain their power, wealth and influence.
5. Fairly wealthy and powerful individuals who, although not evil, wish to retain their power, wealth and influence. e.g. Popes, Bishops, Cardinals, etc.
6. People who are making a good living from religion and also enjoy the prestige which comes from being considered more spiritual than others. e.g. priests, ministers, vicars etc.
7. Well-meaning, but basically powerless, weak and confused religious zealots who seek to acquire a thimble-full of power by converting others.
8. The mass of mindless sheep who unquestioningly support the people in categories 1-7 above.

Scales of Justice

We should refuse to sacrifice our life-energies for such a wasteful and pointless cause as religion, recognizing that if one were to weigh the good against the bad effects of any religion over the last few thousand years, then the scales would come crashing heavily down on the bad side. It would be rather like a one thousand ton weight representing the evil of religion, and a pebble representing the good.

The whole concept of religion represents the exact opposite views of *Fresh Wisdom*.

This is because organized religion is life-debilitating, depressive and looks towards death. We relish life, excitement and joy. We know we will die someday, but we live our life like a warrior until that moment.

Almost all the things which are supposed to bring joy, wonder and excitement to human beings are ruined by the poison of religious thought.

Religion demands that you sacrifice your life's values (money, time, effort) to other people (usually priests) under the disguise of sacrificing them to God.

Religion is, almost by definition, inharmonious due to its divisive nature. You are expected to join one particular group or sect (the only true sect, of course), which then automatically polarizes you against the rest of humanity. Us and them. The rest of humanity are labeled as wrong, evil, sinful, or just misguided, and can only be saved by being converted by you or your group.

Fear is probably the major weapon used by religious con-artists over the centuries. Religious fear is used to ruthlessly cajole the mass of believers into conforming. Fear of damnation, fear of going to hell, fear of judgment day, fear of disapproval by the church, fear of being found out for your sins, fear of the devil, fear of asking questions, fear of the answers, fear of facing your own true thoughts and feelings on a daily basis.

Fresh Thinkers, however, are completely free from fear because we are never immobilized in the present moment. Instead, we live in the present, enjoying each wonderful, spontaneous moment as it unfolds.

Deeply religious people are deeply, soundly asleep. They are not amenable to rational argument. They are not open to logic. They are not prepared to examine the possibility that they are wrong. This is because they are terrified of having their beliefs exposed as beliefs based on man-made rules and regulations.

They have a deep and powerful vested interest in believing their simple fairy tales. The pay-off is comfort and security. Instead of taking refuge in a fairy-tale, we realize there is no one who will make everything alright, and that things never will be alright. This belief empowers us with the knowledge that we have a finite time to live. The result is a happy and guilt-free life, unencumbered by the dead weight of religion.

Religion actively discourages awareness, critical debate or free thought. Any questions which seem a little too searching are met with the response that you must 'have faith' (that is, blind unquestioning belief in something which cannot be proved, and appears to be complete nonsense).

There is even a school of religious thought which states that the more patently ridiculous a fantasy is, then the more *faith* you are showing by believing it. The implication is that the more faith you have (i.e. blind belief in a patent absurdity), then the better a believer you are.

Censorship

Until relatively recently, the flock were not permitted access to written materials concerning their own religion. After all, the con-artists would not like the sheep to actually start studying their religion, or, God forbid, actually questioning the priesthood. The whole point of being a priest is that you control the knowledge, and only dole it out in small handfuls according to your perception of how the sheep will react to this knowledge. The last thing you want is for the sheep to question you, or start thinking for themselves.

Why?

Because the veils which the priests draw across the inner sanctum are exceedingly thin. Too close an inspection might reveal that the altar is bare.[19]

The priests used to be able to rely on the total ignorance and stupidity of the masses. Nowadays they have to rely solely on the latter. Remember that most people were totally illiterate and were incapable of reading the Bible. It is only recently that Catholics (for example) were permitted to read the Bible. Services were, and still are in many places, conducted in Latin - a language completely unknown to the common people. Historically, the church has ruthlessly, repeatedly and deliberately lied to the mass of believers.

They have done this either to blatantly gain advantage for themselves (money, power etc.) or worse, in the belief that these lies were in the best interests of the flock who were considered too vulgar and ignorant to be provided with more accurate information. They considered it best to keep the masses in ignorance.

Organized religion revels in misinformation, illogical thought and downright lies. The vast majority of sheep have absolutely no interest in any aspect of their own religion. They rarely ask questions or enter into debate. Their knowledge of the facts concerning their own religion is virtually nil. In fact they know less about this subject than almost any other subject with which they have had a passing acquaintance. Of course, the reason they do not know is because they

---

[19] The movie *Luther* with Ralph Fiennes is an excellent demonstration of how priests withhold the truth.

do not want to know. They realize, on some level, that their beliefs will not withstand the most cursory examination or questioning and so they adopt a head in the sand attitude and stay that way until they die.

Do Religious Teachers Believe Their Teachings?

It is also a strange fact that many (if not most) priests do not believe more than a small percentage of the 'facts' which they trot out for consumption by the sheep. They continue to support these fabrications for many reasons:

- **Habit**. Even the most arrant nonsense, repeated often enough, will start to sound true. Joseph Goebbels, Stalin, Mao Tse Tung all knew this well.

- **It is a living**. All senior members of the church are making a very comfortable living out of being professional liars. Most of them have a job for life with no threat of redundancy regardless of ability. The con is that the priests are not up-front about their motives, even to themselves. They pretend that making a good living from religion is purely incidental and they are fundamentally interested in helping people. The ranks of the priesthood would rapidly become deserted if the salary was reduced to the level of Social Security, and all possessions were forbidden.

- **Fear**. They fear the consequences of their own questions, and have been trained and conditioned for years to believe that inquisitive thoughts are the devil's work.

- **Simplicity**. They think that the flock would not really understand anything more complex. It is best to repeat a fairy-tale to which their simple minds can relate.

- **Power**. Imagine the power of being a priest. The wonderful feelings of having the masses revere you and fear you. Having people come to you for advice, having them confide their innermost secret thoughts to you. Controlling the lives of the flock. Standing up and lecturing them. The con is that they are not up-front about enjoying this power. Instead they pretend to themselves that this aspect does not interest them and that their only motive is pure self-sacrifice.

- **Superiority**. The priest secretly believes that he is superior to the common herd, and closer to God than they. He fights against this thought, of course, knowing it is wicked and the devil's work - but still he thinks and believes it. He enjoys the masses looking up to him and holding him in great esteem, even awe. He feels a smug sense of goodness, and knows that he will be one of the first in line for a huge, personal thank you from God. He does not like to admit this to himself, of course, and struggles against such wicked, sinful pride, but nevertheless, he feels it. The con is that he pretends (even to himself) not to enjoy the elitist aspect of the job, but to be filled with humility, only performing God's bidding and striving to become the perfect servant of the Lord.

Fresh Thinkers see through all of these things and use them to our advantage. We do not waste life-energy by becoming involved with religion, neither do we seek to convert religious people to our way of thinking. Such a conversion process (if possible) would require an enormous amount of energy.

We are guilt-free in this, because we do not lull people to sleep by poisoning their minds with religious thought - we simply refuse to be lulled ourselves. Neither is it our mission to wake people from their dreams. We are not on any kind of crusade to arouse the masses from their religious slumber.

Seeking The Truth

An interesting example of religious hypocrisy (of which there are countless thousands) is that the majority of believers would state that they are 'seeking the truth'. This is self-deception on their part. They are doing the exact opposite. They would deeply resent the truth if it were presented to them. They would get angry and hot under the collar if the truth were told to them.

The religious masses almost never ask any questions at all about their chosen religion. They certainly do not seek logical answers to reasonable questions. In fact their minds are usually completely closed to new ideas or input. This is the very reason why they joined the group. They want to be controlled and spoon-fed a half-baked version of reality which they can swallow without question. This is comforting for them. The pay-off is security. We, on the other hand, never seek illusory comfort.

Religion offers a pardon for the consequences of your actions as long as you are a good compliant believer. In contrast, we take full responsibility for our every action, and do not seek external beings to take the weight from our shoulders.

Religious Wealth

It is interesting to note that the average so-called Christian in the Western world retains large reserves of wealth while those around him starve to death. An appeal to the sense of fairness offers the religious person absolution for their guilt at this situation. Thus, if they write a $50 check for (say) famine relief, they can feel really good and holy about it for weeks, and not worry too much about the $200,000 of total wealth they have retained for themselves.

Ask any Christian this direct question: "You claim to be a Christian. One of Christ's central teachings is that you have to give up your riches to the poor, and follow Him. While I might accept that this does not mean that you have to walk around in rags and sleep in a ditch, I wonder how you reconcile your alleged Christian beliefs with the fact that your total wealth exceeds $200,000?"

We have never met a Christian who has given up everything and followed Christ. Let us say that again. In a supposedly Christian country, we have never met one single person who has followed Christ's main teaching which was to give up all of your worldly goods, and follow him. Have you ever met such a person?

The best excuse we have heard: "Although I agree that my assets exceed $200,000, I do not really consider that I own them. I long ago gave them to Christ, and I am just waiting for him to tell me what he wants me to do with them all. Meanwhile I consider myself to be merely their guardian." Hmmm...

Are we cold, unfeeling, careless of the starving millions? No. We feel as much as the next person - except that our feelings are genuine because we do not spring from a need for approval, or guilt, or worry, or fear. In fact it might be worth at this point stating our feelings on a particular issue, e.g. the starving millions. Our thoughts are likely to be as follows:

There are hundreds of thousands of causes clamoring for our attention. Everything from wheelchairs for the disabled table tennis team, to the Maori legal fighting fund. The list is almost endless. If we were to start naming these charities at top speed, it would take over four months just to get through the list of names - by which time a hundred new ones will have been formed. Note we are saying nothing whatsoever about the worthiness of these charities.

Our time and funds are limited. If we gave one penny to each of them we would be bankrupt.

It therefore follows that we must strictly limit any charitable giving - preferably to zero.

We are not able to be manipulated by the latest media story, or the church making us feel guilty, or any of the con-artists using any of their weapons.

We are totally guilt-free, and would not feel guilty even if we never gave a penny to any of them - which we rarely do.

We recognize that most charities are limitless sinks of funds and effort. Almost regardless of how many billions are poured in, the problems remain. In fact aid very often causes far more problems than it solves. This is an unpleasant truth to those who seek to absolve their guilt by limited charity.

Finally and vitally: if you and us decide that we will focus our considerable personal power on a (usually very local) charity, then we move into the task with tremendous power, and things really start to happen. We are not talking about a $50 conscience check.

However, we have a policy of non-interference in the lives of others and that means that we rarely become involved in conventional charitable works. The reason is that one can rarely predict the consequences of a so-called good act, and good intentions are simply not enough of an excuse for wholesale interference.

Harmful Charity

Here is just one example of pointless charity - of which there are many thousands. You are probably aware of frequent stories of crop failure, or drought in countries around the world, usually Africa. People are facing starvation almost constantly.

The reason they are starving is because they are struggling to survive on unworkable, worn-out land. A situation which will not improve, only deteriorate. Massive aid has been flown into these desert-like locations, at various points in time. Millions of gallons of drinking water are trucked in. Each operation is paid for by millions of little $50 conscience checks from nice, affluent, middle-class people. Of course, lives are saved in the short-term, but these aid centers act like magnets to hundreds of thousands of people living in outlying districts.

These people are not actually starving, but they are not having too good a time either. So these people from the outlying districts (not the starvation zone) see these aid centers as really great places for a free hand-out to ease their suffering. Unfortunately, this has the effect of displacing large numbers of people from their homes in outlying regions, and attracting them in to an already hopelessly over-populated and worn-out region. This ensures that the death-rate multiplies horribly in successive years when the fuss dies down and the aid workers (and camera crews) leave for the next hot story.

This is an over-simplified example, but the basic message is beware meddling in things about which you know nothing. It is arrogant and dangerous. The motivation is simply one of salving your conscience and justifying the retention of the bulk of your wealth.

Discerning readers do not give possessions or money away to help the poor. However, anyone of any sensitivity must feel something if they are awash with wealth while the rest of the world starves. The difference between a *Fresh Thinker* and the so-called religious person is that:

We are not out to save the world. We realize that it probably cannot be saved anyway. We also realize that so called good actions often only aggravate the problem. Our primary duty is to be happy, and this reflects on others around us. We also know that there is no end to the number of problems around the world. They are limitless.

The religious person does not question the long-term effects of his giving, because his main motivation is to absolve himself from the guilt-feelings caused by his massive retained wealth. So he gives $50 here and there to causes about which he knows little or nothing. He can then put his conscience to sleep for another few months. He neither asks for, nor expects accountability for the aid money. He is not really interested in how the money is spent. He merely wants to know that two points have been added to his 'good boy' total in heaven. He becomes extremely uncomfortable about news stories describing how aid money has been misspent, stolen or squandered. He refuses to listen to these stories. Instead he wants to hear simple little tales of blankets being given to grateful children, or he wants to see a news bite of grinning natives gratefully unloading a few sacks of grain.

Approval

One of the many reasons people follow certain religions is because of approval – an extremely powerful method of influencing the masses.

If the authors feared disapproval, then we would not have included this particular section. It is still very much frowned upon to take such a strong stance against religion. People are very sensitive about their illusions, and they do not like having them exposed.

If you are even a little bit religious, then we are sure you have felt some anger and resentment towards us while reading this section. Not very long ago, we would have been imprisoned, tortured and then murdered in the name of Christ for expressing these thoughts. In those days, the priests held the power of life and death, and they were not squeamish about using those powers.

We consider the comments we have made in this seminar to be fairly mild, just as we consider our comments concerning law and government to be restrained. Why? Because we live in an ultra-repressive society – and it is getting worse. The sheep, of course, believe that they are free and live in a democracy where their vote counts. And enjoy personal power!

If we had confined our comments to certain other religions (which shall remain nameless), then we would have been targeted by fundamentalists, and murdered at the first opportunity. This is not a joke. If we had gone further with our comments concerning government, we would have been listed as dangerous subversives. Our telephones would have a continuous tap on it, mail would be intercepted, bank accounts monitored and possibly we would have been followed to see who we met with.

Many people seek approval through religion. Here are several types of approval:

- **Approval from God**: Most religious people believe in a God who is watching over their every move and smiling in approval at the good things they do, and frowning in disapproval at the naughty things they do. This simplistic view of life relates to childhood, when Mummy and Daddy did exactly this.

- **Approval from the priest**: If you doubt this, simply watch the congregation at the end of a church service. You will see a large group of sycophants swarming around the priest in the hope of getting a quick word of approval from him.

- **Approval from others**: Parading your religion, effectively saying: "Look at me, I'm a really good Christian." Accidentally mentioning the $50 you sent off to Christian Aid last week. Wearing your various badges/poppies/flags which prove what a really caring and wonderful person you are.

- **Approval from your fellow believers**: Joining in the rituals, knowing the new hymn tunes, going to church meetings, being on the committee, doing your bit etc. When you seek the approval of others, you give them power over you to give, or withhold that approval. If they withhold it, you are hurt. If they give it you are like a grateful little doggie, wagging its tail.

Spirituality

Religion has little or nothing to do with true spirituality. It is a man-made system which latches on to people's natural sense of awe, wonder and amazement, just as it exploits their fear of their own mortality and most people who operate the religious con are doing so because they receive a hidden pay-off (the con-artist always gets a pay-off). They are not, in the main, evil people, they are simply con-artists who seek to extract value from you under false pretences. Your pay-off for believing in their nonsense is an illusory comfort and sense of security. You can also feel smug, self-important, chosen and special.

Let us repeat once again, that it is natural to have a feeling of wonder and awe at the amazing mystery of the Universe. It is also natural to speculate upon the origins and purpose of the Universe, and in the microcosm, human existence. We hope that we have not failed in our task of explaining the vast chasm which lies between these natural and wonderful human feelings, and those who seek to prostitute these feelings for their own ends.

What About the Good in Religion?

Finally, we are often confronted with an argument which goes something like this:

"I understand everything you have said, and yes, great evils have been committed in the name of religion, but great good has come too. Most major works of art and music are inspired by religion, and surely if people behave even a little better towards each other as a result of believing in, for the sake of argument, an illusion, then this has got to be good?"

A *Fresh Thinker* answers thus: It is highly likely that an equivalent number of works of art would have been produced without religion. To doubt this is to deny man's basic creativity. You have to imagine Bach, for example, kicking around his house, completely unable to compose because he has never heard of Jesus.

One has to offset religious inspired art against the serious setback to science caused by centuries of religious persecution and suppression of thinking people. Please remember that most art which did not have a religious bias was ruthlessly suppressed by the church. Artists could only get paid for religious works. If they did not turn out such works, they starved. Small wonder that so much art was inspired by religion - it was the only art allowed.

On the second point, we have to disagree. This is effectively the 'happy slave' argument which was current at about the time slavery was abolished. This argument basically stated that there was no point in giving the Negro freedom, or educating them, because they were happy in their ignorance. They did not know any better, so why make them unhappy by telling them about the joys of a free life?

A *Fresh Thinker* rejects this argument outright and believes that human freedom is the ultimate goal. Freedom to be whatever it is you decide to be. Obviously this cannot be achieved if you are a 'happy slave'. This does not mean that we are on a mission to free all slaves (i.e. to wake up the masses); we simply refuse to enslave anyone who comes into contact with us.

To extend this argument to religion, the *Fresh Thinker* believes that it is nice, but irrelevant if some good comes out of believing in a fairy tale. Ancient people believed that sacrificing their children would appease the gods and bring rain, good harvest, fertility, or whatever. No doubt some good came out of this in the form of comfort to the people, but few would argue that belief in such an illusion could be justified by this small amount of good. Some good always results from every act, no matter how evil. This should not be used as a justification for committing evil acts. Hitler, for example, gave us motorways, space rockets and Dad's Army - but this is hardly compensation for the excesses of the Third Reich.

~~~

This section has been contentious for many, and this is because of the deeply ingrained beliefs religion has been responsible for. Many of these beliefs enslave those who have blind faith in their religion. We hope this section has started a process of questioning in your mind. This is an important step before we can move into the really challenging concepts.

There is still much to say on religion, and in a far more positive light.

For now, here is a reminder of the first three of the Immutable Laws of Metaphysical Truths.

1. The Universe and the mind of man were brought into existence out of nothing - or out of something which is currently beyond the ability of our mind to comprehend - by an Initiator outside of this world system.

2. At the Universal Level, there are Two Opposing Forces in existence, and these can be broadly defined as Positive and Negative. The positive force is naturally good, and the negative force is naturally evil. This Opposing Law of Forces is for our personal training in the Management of the Universe.

3. The Negative Force is temporary – with only the Positive Force eventually remaining, resulting in a dimension of Metaphysical Love.

These laws may sound completely foreign to you right now, but rest assured we will be covering them in a subsequent chapter.

~~~

The most beautiful thing we can experience is the mysterious. It is the source of all true art and all science. He to whom this emotion is a stranger, who can no longer pause to wonder and stand rapt in awe, is as good as dead: his eyes are closed. – Albert Einstein

The personal life deeply lived always expands into truths beyond itself. - Anais Nin

The possession of knowledge does not kill the sense of wonder and mystery. There is always more mystery. – Anais Nin

The unique personality which is the real life in me, I can not gain unless I search for the real life, the spiritual quality, in others. I am myself spiritually dead unless I reach out to the fine quality dormant in others. For it is only with the god enthroned in the innermost shrine of the other, that the god hidden in me, will consent to appear.
- Felix Adler, *The Ethical Philosophy of Life*

11. Personal Freedom & Sovereignty

Many readers who have read thus far often think they know it all already, and pride themselves in being relatively free of the system. They smugly sit and read these pages without taking any real action on the material presented, believing that 'it will all be OK' for them.

Well, if you are one of those, it is time for a wake-up call. So here is the next of our controversial statements.

If you are currently contributing to any government taxation program (usually known as Inland Revenue) you are a slave.

If you do not agree with this, then withhold this year's Income Tax and see how long it takes before you are thrown in jail, without a fair trial, without the usual 'innocent until proven guilty' laws applying.

Consider a scale or continuum: At one extreme is *the total slave*; at the other, *the complete Sovereign Individual*.

The total slave is the property of a slave owner. Total slaves do not own their bodies, their time, their labor, nor anything else. Total slaves have no freedom of action; they must do what their masters dictate; they may not do what their masters forbid. They may not own any property whatsoever. Total slaves may be harmed, punished, or killed by their masters without restraint.

Complete Sovereign Individuals, on the other hand, own their own lives, bodies, time, labor, and whatever other property they can practically command, control, or utilize. They have total freedom of action without restraint.

The normal person (whether earning a salary or running their own business) willingly hands over at least fifty percent of their personal wealth in the form of taxes, both as income tax and other hidden taxes like property, fuel, Value Added Tax, etc. This money is handed to other people to spend as they see fit. This person neither asks for, nor expects accountability. They do not know where this money is spent (except in the vaguest way), and they do not care. They do not ask for facts and figures, or expect accountability, honesty or efficiency. If they try to withhold their money, then agents of force will come and take them and throw them in jail.

And the reason for this ludicrous arrangement?

FEAR

The same fear that throughout history has kept slaves returning to their masters to continue working for them.

To convert taxes into time, the average person hands over roughly 20 hours every week (that is nearly 1,000 hours a year) of their precious, limited life to another person, without being paid for it. This is exactly the same life that slaves in recent history endured.

From the government's point of view, their fear keeps them as a nice safe producer/consumer who will not rock the boat too much and will dutifully pay over half of everything they earn in their lifetime to the government. The last thing the government wants is too many financially independent people who are living happy, stress-free and self-fulfilling lives without working too hard.

Why do not they want this? There are many reasons, but here are two for a start:

1. For every one thousand dollars or pounds or whatever currency, the government can legally steal half to play their games with. If you stop paying taxes, they have to stop playing their games.

2. Self-fulfilled and happy people have time to start *thinking*. And when they start thinking they come to many of the conclusions reached in *Fresh Wisdom*. If these conclusions were put into practice by too many people, it would result in severe cut-backs in government power. They do not want that, and so they have a vested interest in keeping you paranoid, afraid, insecure and moderately poor.

Just because you cannot see the slave-chains does not mean they are not there. Chains made of steel are obvious, but chains made of beliefs and fears are not always recognized for what they are.

Many are enslaved because their government can do what they want, take what they want, and individuals cannot refuse. We may have freedom to decide what TV channel to watch tonight (little realizing that the content of every channel is carefully controlled), or just which style of car we will drive to work in, but little power over the rest of our life. Even the home we have worked to pay for over the last decade or more can be taken from us at a moment's notice via 'eminent domain'[20]. Can we refuse? No?

We are thus slaves, living under a dictatorship.

How to Stop Paying Taxes and Claim Back Your Freedom

The purpose of this section is not to convince you to stop paying taxes. We are purely using taxes as a commonly understood mechanism by which many of us are unwittingly enslaved. There are few systems in place which are as commonly understood throughout the world. Taxation is just such a system, easily understood by anyone living in America, England, Australia, Hong Kong, India, Israel, wherever. It is global.

If you are interested in legally opting out of the tax regime in America, consider this:

---

[20] See www.ThreeWorldWars.com/archive/news/real-estate.htm for details.

The US employs a fraudulent taxation system that is completely illegal. Hundreds of thousands have realized this and are quietly withdrawing completely legally from this mass hoax.

In 1986, Roscoe Egger, the IRS Commissioner, publicly admitted that, at that time, thirty five million Americans were no longer filing income tax reports. You can join them, legally, without threat of jail or property confiscation.[21]

You might also be interested in the Canadian situation. On April 22, 2005, a class action suit was filed on behalf of the People of Canada alleging that the Income Tax Act is a fraud.[22]

What is Freedom?

Now that we have established that many of us are in fact slaves, we can progress to discussing what *true* freedom is, and how one can start claiming back that freedom.

First, a look at the Immutable Laws of Freedom and Sovereignty. These Laws are based on:

1. **Privacy**: The ongoing erosion of privacy in the World is the most important issue facing individuals today. Without privacy, we have nothing, or less than nothing. Privacy is a human imperative because privacy of self is an important biological necessity of a sane and stable sense of self. It is a scientific fact that a rational person cannot have their autonomous sense of self (their sense of privacy of self), compromised and still function as a healthy individual. Thinking and creativity require the capacity to make independent judgments. An invasion of our privacy such as that going on in America and other countries today violates that capacity. It is more than important to reclaim our privacy, it is a biological necessity.

2. **Independence**: Only by having money you alone control and having it privately, can one achieve a truly fulfilled life. Offshore money is therefore a pre-requisite to living independently.

3. **Sovereignty**: This is the end ideal to be achieved. A king or queen is not only independent, but also leads their people. In fact they *serve* their people. This is the epitome of success, self-actualization and reaching the Omega Point.

---

[21] http://web.archive.org/web/20041011160453/http://www.solgroup.com/notax/ - The authors are not associated with this group, and you are advised to seek your own advice regarding Income Tax, but it is a route we would seriously consider. The link shown is an archive of a site which is no longer available online.

[22] www.theclassactionsuit.com

The vast majority of people in the world are followers, mere sheep with no particular desire for freedom, nor any wish to be allowed to think for themselves or provide for themselves. They want to have leaders, gurus and to be told exactly what to do and how to think. The majority want someone to take care of them, to make decisions for them and to have the security of belonging to a group, a country, a church, a club that will protect them. They have low levels of self-confidence and a great respect for authority. They have been conned. They do not understand what freedom is, and why it is so important.

Definitions of Freedom

"There is nothing to take a man's freedom away from him, save other men. To be free, a man must be free of his brothers. That is freedom. That and nothing else." [23]

"Full freedom is the absence of restraints, other than natural ones, on an individual's actions. The degree of a man's freedom decreases as the restraints on his actions, beyond those imposed by nature, increase in number or extent. Although the influences reducing a man's freedom can vary in form, the source of any and all such influences can only be the actions of other men." [24]

"Freedom is a condition in which a person's ownership rights in his own body and his legitimate material property are not invaded, are not aggressed against." [25]

"Freedom means self-control; no more, no less." [26]

"It is not recognized in the full amplitude of the word that all freedom is essentially self-liberation - that I can have only so much freedom as I procure for myself by my owness." [27]

"Freedom is living your life as you want to live it." [28]

---

[23] *Anthem* by Ayn Rand, Penguin Books, NY; 1992 - first published in 1938

[24] *Return to Reason: An Introduction to Objectivism* by Paul Lepanto, Exposition Press, NY; 1971

[25] *For a New Liberty: The Libertarian Manifesto* by Murray N. Rothbard, Collier Books, NY; 1978 - first published 1973

[26] *The Discovery of Freedom: Man's Struggle Against Authority* by Rose Wilder Lane, Arno Press & The New York Times, NY; 1972 - first published in 1943

[27] *The Ego & Its Own: The Case of the Individual Against Authority* by Max Stirner, Rebel Press, London; 1982 - first published in German in 1845 as *Der Einzige und sein Eigentum*

[28] *How I Found Freedom in an Unfree World* by Harry Browne, Avon Books, NY; 1973

Now we are getting to the core of what *Fresh Wisdom* is all about. The concept is a coherent philosophy, a plan for a stress free, healthy, prosperous life not limited by government interference, the threat of nuclear war, the reality of food and water contamination, litigation, domestic conflicts, taxation, persecution or harassment. Whether your concern may be the increasing drumbeat of war, a domestic issue which appears expensive to resolve, or an unwarranted accusation by some Gestapo-style government agency, *Fresh Wisdom* offers escape. It is a way out of any negative situation created and imposed upon you by any external entity. Many individuals choose to vent their frustrations with acts of violence. The *Fresh Thinker* merely avoids conflict by refusing to play where the rules are unfair.

What we are doing in these pages is conditioning and training our mind to unlearn all the beliefs instilled in us from birth, which entrap us. This is true freedom. This is the ultimate "Aha!" experience.

With the *Fresh Wisdom* philosophy, you will be able to remain comfortably beyond the reach of Big Brother's (or anyone else's) ever extending grasp. It is impossible for any government to attack or wipe out *Fresh Thinkers* because we are an amorphous group without consistent behavior patterns. We cannot be identified, classified or isolated from the general run of sheep. Thus, unlike some publicity seeking individualists or tax rebels, we court no danger and invite no confrontations.

Ultimate Freedom

As *Fresh Thinkers*, only restrictions imposed by ourselves can keep us from experiencing the wonders of the world. We can and will drive, fly or sail across international frontiers when and where we want, alone or with anyone we choose. We are mentally, financially and physically prepared to leave anywhere we happen to be and go to the other end of the earth at the first whiff of danger or just in search of greener pastures. We are able to move fast and decisively, to disappear and resurface anywhere, anytime.

We can read what we want to read, eat what we want to eat, see what we wish to see, imbibe or ingest as desired and invest anywhere in anything. We are completely free from restrictions placed upon us by governments. We can buy or sell what we please. We can associate with, employ or live with people whom we find agreeable and pleasing. If we want to change friends, employment or climate for any reason, we can do so almost instantaneously without the need to get any sort of permission from the state.

Until we adopt this mode of thinking, the range of opportunities denied to us is inconceivable. We do not miss the things of which we are unaware. This manual may raise your consciousness as to the true nature of freedom. It is one way to rid one's self of limitations.

We are able to study any philosophy, raise and educate our children in our beliefs and opinions without contradiction from our government-controlled school curriculum. We need not follow the dictates of an obtuse school commissar who bans our favorite books and forbids mention of those truths we find most self-evident.

We finally become able to invent, improvise, abandon, reject or follow any religion, personal morality or way of life we choose. We can shop, have a drink or eat when we want, not just when the local laws allow restaurants and stores to be open. For those with unconventional thoughts, habits or beliefs, the *Fresh Wisdom* philosophy is the answer. Life can be lived spontaneously, free, without state imposed restrictions. Becoming a *Fresh Thinker* means never again having to ask permission or submit to any higher authority. Life is free of permits, licenses, exit permits, visas, currency restrictions, taxes, record keeping, bureaucrats, social workers, litigation, filing and reports.

We need not put up with rules, regulations or laws we find personally offensive, inconvenient or immoral. Thus if it suits us, without any government or church dispensation, we may have as many spouse-equivalents as are desired. The range of possibilities for greater freedom is expanded to whatever can be conceived. We may be celibate and need not own a car or acquire any other status symbol unless so desired.

On the other hand, the *Fresh Thinker* can live in a highly controlled society if they so choose, if for some reason this sort of community gives them a sense of security or perhaps even superiority. This is all about options. The more options one has, the more free that individual becomes. We can live under whichever system suits us best.

This freedom, however, does not mean that we should be or can be irresponsible by causing problems, injury or pain to others. The message is not to encourage greed, lust, irresponsibility, immorality or any of the other seven deadly sins.[29] On the contrary, to avoid government's heavy hand is to avoid violating local laws and morality. We must go physically to those places where doing what we want to do is accepted as ordinary behavior. There is no point in spending time where our lifestyle, appearance or conduct will cause moral offense or get us into difficulties with local authorities. This way of life involves

[29] www.whitestonejournal.com/seven/

discovering those places where your particular pleasures are legal and accepted.

This is Ultimate Freedom – breaking free from any and all previously held belief systems, and living life the way it was *meant* to be lived.

The Freedom Lifestyle

Once again, we are getting a little ahead of ourselves. We are talking about physically moving somewhere, when we know this may not be possible for some right now, for a variety of reasons. All we really want to cover for now is preparing oneself mentally to break free from limiting beliefs.

~~~

> Side Note: There is a very real reason why we speak about relocating away from a densely populated city, ideally before mid-2007. For more information about the real state of the world militarily and economically and how you can prepare for what appears to be the coming World War 3, see www.threeworldwars.com.

~~~

As a final note on this topic, it is really not as expensive as most believe to be able to leave your comfortable home in a Western nation to lead a truly free life. As a rough rule of thumb, you need approximately fifteen times your desired annual salary 'in the bank' if you are to give up working for a living. For example, if you decide that you need $20,000 gross every year to sustain your chosen life-style, then you will need fifteen times this amount, or $300,000 invested to allow you to draw your chosen salary, and leave the capital reasonably inflation-proof.

If you only need $10,000 gross, then you will require $150,000 invested.

The very best state to be in, concerning money, is one of total fearlessness, because if you are fearful, then other people will use fear to control your behavior. If jobs are short, then they will use your fear of poverty to extract all sorts of extra values from you. This might mean that you have to work harder for less pay, or touch your cap a bit more respectfully when the boss comes in.

Money & Achieving Fearlessness

The advanced *Fresh Thinker* has enough money so that they need not work if they decide not to. In practice, they often continue to work at some level for the challenge or sheer enjoyment, but they are not dependent upon this generated income.

There is a second, and more important aspect to the fearlessness of a *Fresh Thinker*. Because they enjoy health, wealth and freedom, they genuinely would not care if some terrible disaster reduced them to a humble life of basic existence (similar to a monk in a monastery). It is highly characteristic of our behavior that we win in every situation, so we would view our reduction to absolute poverty as a great chance to catch up on meditations concerning the deeper meaning of life, or some other philosophical activities.

The *Fresh Thinker* would far rather be wealthy than poor, but if riches were denied, then we would still be happy being poor.

In order to become a true free thinking individual, you must be prepared, in principle at least, to become totally poor. Why?

Because if you are at least prepared for this possibility, then you do not fear it. You might not like it, but you do not fear it.

Fear Of Poverty

Fear of poverty in the sheep is the major source of their lack of personal power. One cannot have personal power if one allows other people to dictate to you exactly what to do with most of one's waking time - and yet this is exactly what most people in employment do. They fear poverty and so they stay in jobs which they do not enjoy, as wage-slaves, working for bosses who use fear to manipulate them.

Bosses and the government actually want the population to be in a state of semi-panic concerning unemployment and the economy. Why?

Because bosses and the government want the population to work as hard as possible for the absolute minimum reward. This scenario brings in maximum money and personal power for those in charge, and prevents the masses from waking up.

Most bosses secretly long to have queues of people clamoring at the factory gates for the chance of a job, because this means that they can pick the very best people, pay them almost nothing, and command absolute loyalty, obedience and respect from them.

Likewise, the government desires the same thing, as this keeps inflation way, way down, and ensures that the masses devote 101% of their waking time to slaving in order to earn a crust. No time is then left for thinking, questioning or rebelling.

The opposite scenario - the one detested by governments and bosses alike - is one where the country is in full employment. When jobs are in plentiful supply, companies simply cannot hire staff because no-one is available. Wage prices soar, bringing steep inflation; companies are forced to hire third and fourth-rate employees, and bosses become fearful that their employees will simply up and leave at the slightest provocation, to be snapped-up by one of a hundred rival companies all desperate for workers. Employees, on the other hand, are not fearful since they know that they could have their pick of a hundred different jobs. Bosses then actually have to start being nice to their workers in an effort to keep them.

From the government's point of view, when the country is in full employment, millions of people start working part-time (for full-time money) or giving up work altogether. This gives them time to think and to work out what they really want from their lives. They might actually start to become happy and self-fulfilled, even, heaven forbid......*content*!

Is it starting to make sense now why there is such high unemployment in your country?

People enjoying new-found freedom, start to question all sorts of things which they had been too busy to even think about in leaner times; furthermore, they do not consume so much (happy, contented people tend to consume far less than unhappy, trapped people), which has the effect of making them less able to be manipulated by adverts, greed, worry, etc.

Freeing Yourself From Poverty

Fresh Thinkers use several techniques for freeing themselves from fear of poverty:
- Become completely and utterly debt-free (including mortgage).
- Maximize personal income.
- Minimize outgoings (expenditure).
- Minimize or reduce to zero responsibilities to support others financially.
- Start an independent business.

Advanced *Fresh Thinkers* have taken these five steps. The result is that they have absolutely no financial concerns of any description. This does not mean that they are all millionaires (although many of them are very wealthy). They take the required steps in their lives to ensure that their income exceeds their outgoings.

Please re-read the above sentence at least three times, as this simple statement conceals a profound principle of becoming solvent. Notice we are saying *solvent* and not wealthy. Solvent means that your income exceeds your outgoings, and so, by definition, you are becoming steadily richer.

In contrast, if your outgoings exceed your income, then you are slipping further into debt with every day that passes.

This trivial observation is at the absolute heart of becoming first debt-free, and then solvent, yet remarkably few people apply this simple fact to their own financial situation. They tend to think that it is much, much more complicated than that - it is not.

The aspiring *Fresh Thinker* should immediately take two vital steps:

- Increase their income.
- Greatly reduce their outgoings.

All *Fresh Thinkers* must do this until their income exceeds their outgoings. This single step confers unimaginable personal power as one starts to shrug off the burden of debt and insolvency.

Overcoming fear is largely a question of having the correct attitude. You must also have the desire, even hunger, to seize personal power. Once you decide that you are no longer going to live in fear of money, certain things automatically follow.

1. You take steps to become completely debt-free (this includes paying off your mortgage if you have one). If you are in debt, even by a small amount, then you are forced to spend a certain amount of your time working to service this debt. If you lose your job, then you cannot pay your debts and certain penalties will come into play (e.g. losing your house). It is fear of these penalties which keeps you locked into the work cycle.

2. You take the required steps to maximize income and minimize outgoings. Why? Because you realize that the route to solvency and eventual wealth is through ensuring that your income exceeds your outgoings. Simple, but so very, very true.

3. You take steps to remove 'freeloaders' from your 'payroll'. Other people can be a huge drain on your resources. People are fundamentally lazy and do not (quite rightly) want to work eight hours a day in some mindlessly tedious job. If they can get someone else (i.e. you) to foot the bill while they sit at home having a relatively easy life, then they will - particularly if you allow them. The *Fresh Thinker* has cut all excess financial encumberments from their life.

4. You take steps to leave full-time employment and start your own business. Why? Because only by working for yourself can you:
   - Command a far higher salary than is available in any similar paid employment.
   - Be in control of your own destiny.
   - Have a shot at becoming seriously wealthy.

~~~

A short note about debt: Debt, when handled correctly, can be a useful way of increasing liquidity. However, the sheep seldom understand the workings of debt, and the consequences when debt becomes unmanageable. We would encourage to use debt wisely and to your advantages, but only within a framework of being otherwise debt free.

In other words, never rely on debt, including a mortgage for your house or a lease for your car.

~~~

We have wandered from the subject of Freedom somewhat, but only indirectly. A *Fresh Thinker* has taken all four of the steps discussed above, with the result that they are totally fearless concerning money. This confers a huge amount of personal power and freedom to them, as money (or rather lack thereof) is the number one illusion used to control the masses.

To finally get back to what *Fresh Wisdom* is all about. Our methodology consists of the practical knowledge, methods, and skills to live free in an unfree world. This could be called the "Harry Browne" principle as expounded in his book *How I Found Freedom in an Unfree World.*[30] *Fresh Wisdom* enables you to run rings around terrocrats (any individual or entity intent on destroying your personal freedom). *Fresh Wisdom*, properly applied, enables you to lawfully, legally, elegantly, and safely exit terrocrat systems. It also enables you to protect your earnings and assets from the marauding ravages of terrocrats. In short, *Fresh Wisdom* allows you to live life according to your rules, while being cognizant of, and side-stepping rules that you do not wish to follow.

Now perhaps you can understand why *Fresh Wisdom* is not for the sheeple. Very few can handle the responsibility of making their own rules. We are not for a minute suggesting anarchy – we are suggesting a sensible, carefully thought through set of life values and principles, which lead to a fulfilled life.

What is Sovereignty?

The idea of a Free Sovereign Individual and what you have to do to become free, is a process, and not something that can be achieved by just anyone. In some very important aspects a Free Sovereign Individual is a special breed of human. Listed below are the basic assumptions, assertions, or affirmations that a Free Sovereign Individual lives by:

- I am free;
- I own myself (I am sovereign);
- I am responsible;
- I choose the values by which I live;
- I live my life the way I want to;
- I practice association by consent;

---

[30] *How I Found Freedom in an Unfree World* by Harry Browne (Avon Books, NY; 1973)

- I want others to enjoy the same freedom.

Implications of Sovereignty

Each Free Sovereign Individual has his or her own set of basic assumptions, whether explicitly formulated or not. Some of the implications of the assumptions listed previously are covered in this section, with thanks to Frederick Mann. [31]

I Am Free

One cannot become free by merely asserting that you are free. It is very difficult for people who have not lived free to discover that they are free. But people can discover that they control their energy, and that - ultimately - every action they take follows from a decision in their brain. Reading *The Discovery of Freedom* by Rose Wilder Lane may assist this discovery.

> *My mind and my body are in my power... Whatever beliefs I might have about not being free are beliefs in my mind. I chose those beliefs. I can change those beliefs.*

I Own Myself (I Am Sovereign)

Either you own yourself, or somebody else owns you and you are a slave. By extension, if you own yourself, you own your life, your mind, your body, your property, and the fruit of your labor. Being sovereign and owning yourself are the same thing.

The discovery that you are sovereign also follows from the realization that you are free and that all coercive political systems on planet earth today are fraudulent hoaxes. Reading *The Constitution of No Authority*[32] may assist this discovery.

> *I do not rule others, nor am I ruled by others. I am sovereign over my life, mind, body, and property.*

I Am Responsible

The realization that you are responsible follows from an increasing awareness of the links between your actions (and non-actions) and their consequences. Your choices have consequences. The kind of life you now lead, your degree of freedom, and the state of your health are consequences of your choices. You have created your life. You are responsible, whether you know it or not.

> *To a very large extent, I cause my actions, I produce my own outcomes, and I determine what happens to me. Though I*

---

[31] www.BuildFreedom.com - © Copyright 1994 Terra Libra. Used with permission.
[32] www.buildfreedom.com/tl/tl07.shtml

realize that while I am free to choose my actions, I am not free to choose the consequences of my actions.

Being responsible also means that I keep the agreements I make.

I Choose the Values by Which I Live

Whatever moral code you live by, you chose it - even if by default. If you decide to live by the "laws of a country" (so-called), that is your choice. A Free Sovereign Individual knows that there can be as many moral codes as there are conscious individuals.

I Live My Life the Way I Want To

For the most part, this is really an obvious statement of fact. To think otherwise is to deceive yourself. If you wanted your life to be different you would have created it differently through your choices. Of course, we do realize that "chance events" have considerable influence - but it is the victim or slave mentality who blames external factors and feigns helplessness.

I Practice Association by Consent

Force or coercion by human against human is a remnant of the practice of slavery. I believe in voluntary association. I do not force or coerce others. I organize my life so as to reduce coercion from others against me to a minimum.

I Want Others to Enjoy the Same Freedom

Other Free Sovereign Individuals enrich my life. Social contact with them tends to be rewarding, business mutually profitable. In general, life is more fun and rewarding among a circle of Free Sovereign Individuals. Benefits result from my successful attempts to assist others to increase their freedom.

Parallel: A rational person seeks associations with other rational individuals, and profits from their existence through voluntary exchange in which all parties gain value.

Seize Your Freedom!

(This section is based on a flyer written by the mysterious author "J.E.T.")

So you want to be free? Then become free. All the freedom is yours which you are able to seize. How do you seize freedom? By avoiding, evading, escaping, discouraging, overpowering, destroying, or otherwise frustrating anyone who initiates force, fraud, or the threat of force against you.

Do you beg for freedom? - "But the oppressors ignore my pleas for freedom," you complain. Do you expect them to set you free? (Graffiti in a Las Vegas shopping mall: SLAVES NEED MASTERS.) As you yourself point out, your oppressors have the morals which would shame a beast of the forests. As long as you obey their rules, no matter how onerous, and pay their taxes, no matter how burdensome - why should they set you free? - Why should they relinquish the easy life of a parasite?

"And the oppressors dupe my neighbors who are confused, unaware, and apathetic," you protest. Do you expect them not to deceive? - Not to tame their flocks? The herdsman can milk only tame cows; the shearer can shear only submissive sheep; the tyrant can drive only obedient slaves...

"We must overturn the oppressors," some of you proclaim, "and rule wisely and justly in their place." Then go do it - if you can. But do not be surprised when the oppressors stampede their bewildered subjects against you.

"We must educate - teach increasing numbers our values and ideas," others shout, "And some day truth will prevail and evil will be banished from the earth." But as even you admit in your more reflective moments, this will take time - much time. So how shall you live the only life you will ever have? And how many followers can you attract and hold if you offer only visions of a paradise for their great grandchildren?

"I do want freedom," you cry, "But there is no way to get it now - no chance to elect, no means to revolt, and no place to go." I reply: If you want freedom, seize it.

"But my oppressors are organized into a powerful government, an omnipotent state - their laws shackle me," you object, "And they have thousands of agents and millions of police." I reply: However, each of their minions has only the same two eyes, the same two hands, and usually not as much brains as you or I. They are individuals. They cannot be everywhere. They cannot see everything. They cannot understand everything. They cannot do everything. You do not have to obey them.

"But they collect a tax on my earnings before I even see it," you protest. Only if you are so craven as to hand it over. Discover ways to avoid their extortions: Get your earnings under your own control; trade with those who practice freedom; or be a Gypsy who sells - and flees.

"But they will confiscate my property," you quaver. Only if you are so foolish as to lead them to it. Convert your wealth into forms you can conceal. Put it where they cannot get at it. And rent your shops and homes - or mortgage them to the hilt.

"But they will throw me in jail," you object. Only if you are so careless as to stumble over them - they who have trouble apprehending morons and psychopaths. Make yourself difficult to find.

"But that is too much trouble," you complain, "I would rather follow their rules and pay their taxes - lick their boots and hone their axes - do everything they demand - and maybe, oh maybe, they will leave me alone just a little." Then tag along with the sheep to slaughter, you who expect freedom on a silver platter. For how long can you appease the tyrant who will demand more and more, until he owns you completely?

And what do we know of this libertarian utopia that some of you dream of? In every land of which we hear, there are some who covet the lives and creations of others - predators who rob and enslave the weak, the foolish, and the cowardly. And when have they failed to recruit millions to vote for them, finance them, and work for them as humble agents and police?

Some predators prowl alone or in small gangs, slinking about as criminals. So the Free Sovereign Individuals go about like tigers - armed and ready for self-defense.

Some predators join together, masquerading and strutting about as "rulers." So the Free Sovereign Individuals go about like foxes - inconspicuous and ready to hide.

In almost every land, those with the courage to assert their freedom seldom need to fight or hide - for the predators live off the easy prey.

Now, at last, I have the key –
The elixir of liberty –
For the first time in history –
And once sufficient numbers see...
All the freedom is yours which you are able to seize. [33]

~~~

Side Note: An excellent table showing the difference between the Republic of the United States and the modern day Corporation it has become can be found here: www.worldnewsstand.net/guns/truth.htm. The table explains clearly what this means to your personal sovereignty.

An extensive list of freedom related reading material to educate yourself on your rights as a Sovereign Individual can be found here: www.wealth4freedom.com/truth/links2educate.htm

---

[33] www.buildfreedom.com/selflib.htm

12. The Fresh Wisdom Ethos

We have covered much ground since we started. Perhaps you are one of the few who became a little frustrated with some of the lessons, wondering when we were going to get into the real meat. This is that point in time. Your patience is about to be rewarded.

This is a very important chapter because we are going to answer questions which may have been plaguing you:

- What is Freedom Technology's real agenda with *Fresh Wisdom*?
- If people do not generally have my best interests at heart, how is Freedom Technology any different - why should they just want to help someone for no reason?
- The authors slated religion in Chapter 10, and yet they make mention of a Creator – what's up with that? How is it possible to teach me how to have a successful, happy life without promoting some type of religion or political belief?
- The authors have consistently said that not all people are equal, that some are sheep. And yet the U.S. Constitution says that "All men are created equal and are endowed by their Creator with certain inalienable rights...". The Bible also says that all men are created equal in God's eyes. Why should I believe the authors when it goes against what the U.S. Constitution and the Bible says?
- The authors have a selfish motive for promoting their particular philosophy of life – what is that motive?

These are all excellent questions, which we are not going to answer immediately, but by the end of this chapter you will have understood why these questions do not faze us in the least. In fact, the very fact that you may be asking these questions (as others have) prove to us that you are still enslaved by certain belief systems which are holding you back, and we still have some work to do to break them.

For those who found the previous chapters a little *obvious*, we are pleased you stuck with us and understood that we had to lay the foundations. We had to explain that everyone (even you, and yes, even us) have paradigms which have been conditioned into our thinking. Remember the first lesson with the picture of the old and young woman? Ten seconds of conditioning affected the way the composite picture was interpreted. A lifetime of conditioning affects our paradigm – our world view – or the way in which we interpret what's happening in the world around us.

In this chapter we are going to answer the questions above and explain our paradigm, which is built on empirically proven scientific means, not the myths and the ravings of 'gurus'. By the end of this chapter you will be able to fully judge whether the philosophy of *Fresh Wisdom* makes sense to you. Some of these teachings will be difficult for you to accept. If they are, it is not because the teachings are wrong (we will prove this to you) – it is because your existing paradigm is still limiting you. And we understand how difficult this may be to accept, hence the introductory foundation which we have been building since explaining *paradigm shifts*.

Basic Axioms

Before we explain our paradigm, let us list a number of givens that we have covered in earlier chapters, either directly or indirectly. If you cannot yet accept these givens, perhaps you should re-read the relevant chapter. You will have a difficult time accepting our paradigms if we cannot treat the following axioms as absolutely given and accepted – no further discussion required.

Axiom #1 – Reducing Controls

In order to become free, *Fresh Thinkers* greatly reduce the external controls placed on their life. They will not allow themselves to be controlled by anyone (including Freedom Technology and the authors of *Fresh Wisdom*). They recognize the various controlling tactics for what they are, and will not allow them to influence their life negatively. These people and institutions are referred to as Controlling Artists, or Con Artists. *Fresh Thinkers* understand that these Controlling Artists have a vested interest in trying to control them.

Axiom #2 – Avoid Con Artists

Con artists seek to maximize the volume of life's pleasures which flow their way, by conning money, energy, time and talent from other people. By bending the talents, energy and time of the mass of people to their will, such individuals and organizations seek to profit with minimum effort on their part. *Fresh Thinkers* understand this and avoid Con Artists.

Axiom #3 – Recognizing Illusions

Fresh Thinkers make it a lifelong task to continually unmask the illusions created by others. The extent to which they believe in one or more of the illusions is the extent to which they are still enslaved. The facets of life which are home to the greatest number of illusions are:
1. Health and Longevity
2. Relationships and Romantic Love
3. Religion
4. Finance, Money and Wealth Creation
5. Personal Freedom

There are, of course, many other minor illusions, but your knowledge of the five main categories of illusions will provide you with the information required to tackle the smaller and less significant ones. Remember – the illusions are the vehicles which people who want something from you use to extract your time, money and talents.

Axiom #4 – All Are Not Equal

Very few people will choose the path of freedom and unlimited personal power in their lives. In this respect, all are created equal in the options available to them, but not all make the same (equal) choices in life.

As *Fresh Thinkers*, we recognize this inequality, and will not attempt to convince the sheep of the value of this lifestyle. We realize this is an impossible and thankless task.

Axiom #5 – Altruism

True altruism does exist, but is so rare that it can be ignored for all intents and purposes. By true altruism, we mean an act which is entirely selfless with absolutely no pay-off of any description.

Altruistic acts do not always achieve a positive effect on humanity, as the help provided is often misguided and harmful.

Altruism is used by Con Artists to exploit your natural and normal human desire to assist others. They turn this desire to their benefit by getting you to sacrifice your time, money and talents to them by pretending to be needy, or pretending to act altruistically, while obtaining a secret pay-off.

Axiom #6 – Rules and Regulations

Fresh Thinkers live by their own set of rational, coherent and internally generated rules, which may, or may not agree with the externally imposed laws. Sometimes they will, sometimes they will not. They follow these regulations and accept full and total responsibility for their every action. They also accept the consequences on a strict cause and effect basis, if these actions happen to conflict with the law of the land at a particular time, and in a particular place. We have no opinion on the fairness of any particular law, since we know that all laws are more or less arbitrary and 'unfair'.

Example: When in a foreign country where the known penalty for smuggling drugs is death, then we would not be surprised at the penalty imposed if we were caught smuggling drugs.

Axiom #7 – Fairness

The world is, and always has been, an unfair place. *Fresh Thinkers* know this, and do not find it surprising. They do not squander their life-energies in an attempt to change this situation.

The statement "It is not fair!" comes only from the mouth of a sheep that is controlled by the law, and is whining because the rules are not tight enough. Someone has slipped through the net, and the sheep want the net closed.

Throughout history, innocent men and women have been imprisoned, tortured and beaten-up or killed by the state under various disguises - and it is still happening today. Is it fair? No. Is the law fair? No. Does a *Fresh Thinker* expect it to be fair? No.

Axiom #8 – Purpose

The uninitiated masses almost never know their real reasons for doing anything. The vast majority know almost nothing whatsoever about the mechanism of government, and yet they continue to vote and pay taxes. The vast majority know almost nothing whatsoever about Spiritual Truths, and yet they continue to support their chosen religion, without ever investigating other belief systems. *Fresh Thinkers*, in contrast, never accept anything without questioning and understanding it. They also understand that their life has a purpose, even though their purpose may not yet have been fully defined or understood.

Axiom #9 – Religion

Religions and cults are man-made inventions designed to allow an elitist priesthood to con value out of those that follow them. *Fresh Thinkers* do not blindly follow any man-made religion.

Axiom #10 – Morality

Conventional morals are purely influenced by the latitude and longitude at which you happen to find yourself, together with the date currently showing on your calendar. In other words, laws are applicable to the country you happen to be in at a specific time. It is likely that those laws were different in the past and do not currently apply to other locations. This means that conventional morality is based on arbitrary, man-made, fickle laws. The morals of a *Fresh Thinker* are not based on man-made laws but are instead internally generated, according to the Immutable Laws of Nature.

Axiom #11 – Responsibility

Responsibility for what happens in the life of a *Fresh Thinker* rests solely with that person. This is particularly true when known laws are transgressed, and we do not question the fairness or otherwise of the consequences.

Axiom #12 – Relationships

Successful relationships hinge upon a continued and approximately equal exchange of values between the partners. When an imbalance occurs a *Fresh Thinker* either addresses the imbalance or ends the relationship.

The Freedom Technology Mission Statement

Now that we have discussed and exposed many of the illusions the sheep are enslaved by, we are finally free to progress to the meat of *Fresh Wisdom*. At this point we are able to expose our reason for making this information available – our Mission Statement if you will.

Stimulate Creativity

We want to open eyes – to stimulate independent thought. We want every *Fresh Thinker* to think for themselves, unlike the sheep that are spoon-fed and hence indoctrinated.

Years of exposure to the media, and more recently the Internet, have stifled creative thought because of the lack of stimulating content. The books on best seller lists, the entertainment broadcast on TV, the 'life-changing' advice presented in glossy magazines are all merely rehashed fillers, providing no real mental stimulation. No wonder the sheep are in the state they are in.

Opposing Forces

We want to help *Fresh Thinkers* discover or become aware of the fact that there are 2 forces at work: positive and negative; light and darkness; love and life, hate and death; yin and yang. While this appears to be a statement of the obvious, we then wish to show how most people are subject to the negative force (no matter how enlightened they may think they are). And finally, we want to show how to turn fully and meaningfully from the negative force to the other.

Guilt

We want to make *Fresh Thinkers* aware of the amount of guilt that enslaves us all and how to deal with it. To some extent we have covered most of that in preceding chapters, but there is still more to come. We want to get this guilt cleared up once and for all, freeing us to higher levels of spiritual awareness and performance.

Purpose

We want to reveal the ultimate potential and purpose for each life. We want to prove empirically that there is not just a black hole of nothing at the end, but a significantly (mind-bogglingly) higher existence after this one, in another dimension. We are not referring to a dimension filled with aliens, shape-shifters and the like. We refer to that dimension as the Quantum Spectrum or E5, and we will explain this all in due course.

We want to enable motivated individuals to recognize that there is a Purpose to their individual life and that any effort exerted now *will* yield unimaginable rewards, making this present life meaningful to the extreme.

Provable Reality

We are fully aware of the multitude of already existing writings that cover similar material: Self Help Books, Spiritual Empowerment Books, and the list goes on. But we wish to demonstrate this (The Quantum Spectrum) empirically, by employing measurable and provable scientific means. In our view, the vast majority of writings on this subject to date are based upon myths and the ravings of self-proclaimed 'gurus', who achieve nothing more than give their readers mental constipation.

In Control

We want to free people from enslavement to traditions, systems and propaganda. The alternative is enlightenment, freedom, understanding and incredible power, in which they are in control of their own life and destiny. You have seen the results of some of this in previous chapters, with much more still to come.

Omega Point

We want to enable *Fresh Thinkers* to reach their own personal Omega Point of ultimate understanding of life, the Universe and beyond.

What We Are Not

We have introduced a number of new terms, and now might be an appropriate moment to set your mind at rest about what we are not trying to achieve.

We are not trying to control you (Axiom 1). You are free to draw your own conclusions about the material we present. We frequently challenge and remind you to listen for the ring of truth.

We are not Con Artists (Axiom 2). By the end of this chapter you will have zero doubt about our agenda, or our motivation for making this material available.

We are not presenting yet another illusion (Axiom 3). We will refer you to the empirical proof for anything that requires it (as supplemental reading, otherwise this manual would easily turn into 20 years of reading.)

We know that this material is not meant for everyone (Axiom 4), so we will never force you to accept anything. You are encouraged at all stages to critically analyze any theory we present.

We are not a charity, and nor are we presenting this material as an entirely selfless act (Axiom 5). We will explain the value exchange we are expecting soon.

We impose absolutely no rules and regulations on you (Axiom 6). You are free to lead your life exactly as you please. We would be surprised if your life did not change as a result of completing this manual, but we never dictate any specific action.

We are not trying to make the world a better place, or make it fairer (Axiom 7). This is an impossible task, and not one we would ever consider undertaking.

We will not define your life purpose (Axiom 8). What you choose to do with this material, and your life, is entirely up to you.

Although we will discuss many matters of a spiritual nature, we are not a religion. Nor are we a cult (Axiom 9). Both cults and religions extract time, talents and money from you under false pretenses. We will not insult your intelligence and destroy your life by doing the same.

We are not about to impose a moral code on you (Axiom 10). The moral code by which you choose to live your life is totally under your control.

The people behind Freedom Technology are not legal experts, medical professionals, ministers of religion, investment advisors or licensed counselors and shall not accept liability or responsibility to any person (Axiom 11). Therefore, you release Freedom Technology from any responsibility for any actions you take as a result of strategies you learn here. You agree that you are solely responsible for seeking the necessary professional advice before implementing any of the strategies we teach.

The concept of Freedom Technology is not easy to express in a succinct manner, an Elevator Speech, if you will. We hope however that the explanation of what we are not has cleared up any reservations you may have about continuing this journey with us.

The Basis of a World View

A consistent, stable, valid and workable World View should be able to provide reasonable and believable answers to at least 4 aspects:

1. How the Universe came about;
2. The nature and purpose of Man;
3. Good and Evil: How to resolve the inherent conflicts in the 'evil' Nature of Man with supposed 'goodness'. In other words, how to bridge the gap between the expected goodness of Man and the evidenced evil behavior so prevalent in society;
4. The Future: Are we to accept Nihilism (a black hole of nothingness) or is there an explanation of any existence after this dimension.

Before we explain our World View, we require a brief explanation of a few terms we are about to introduce.

The present dimension in which the material Universe exists consists of four dimensions:

1. Length,
2. Breadth,
3. Height and
4. Time.

All matter exists in this dimension at a particular point and time. Since there are 4 dimensions limiting all existence, we will refer to this dimension as *E4*.

The next dimension, in which Time is no longer a limiting factor (Eternity), and which scientists commonly refer to as the Quantum Spectrum, is therefore called E5.

This dimension is also called *heaven* by many religions (who do not understand the scientific basis of E5).

The Biblical World View

At this point we must ask you to hold judgment based on any preconceived religious (including atheist) beliefs you may or may not have. Remember that we are trying to break free from pre-implanted paradigms.

The Biblical World View is the only scientifically (empirically) provable, sustainable and viable World View that has no inconsistencies. It is for this reason that we have chosen the Biblical World View on which to base these premises. Note that these are not Christian, Catholic, Protestant or any other religion's World View – it is a Biblical World View, which can be defined as follows (answering the 4 aspects raised previously).

1. The Universe was created by an Outside-Of-This-System Initiator at a specific point and identifiable time, in keeping with known laws which are currently in use to determine things like space trajectories of interplanetary craft, microwave transmissions, etc.

2. The purpose for which Man was also created and put into this System is for training: Training in understanding of the Universe and dealing with the 2 forces of positive and negative that are inherent in the system, commonly called 'good' and 'evil'. An additional purpose is for future E5 Management Tasks - we will have specific jobs in the next dimension.

3. The solution for this good and evil or positive/negative conflict is provided by Initiator. The resolution of the problem of the existence of 'evil' is not achieved by Man, but supplied extraneously (from outside the system) by Initiator. Recognition of this is part of the training and comes for all at some point. For some it is given to them to understand now in the E4 and for the others, it will be given later in E5. In other words: *all* people will eventually understand fully, when (in Initiator's own time) their eyes are opened by Initiator (and no-one else, although humans can plant seeds).

4. The Future: There is another (provable) Dimension (E5) in which Time is not a limiting factor. All human beings do appear into this dimension – it is an inherent (automatic) outcome of the Created Order. This present order is merely an interim state of preparation; similar to the birth of a child after being nurtured in the womb (E4) and coming into the world (E5). It can also be equated with the symbolism of the classic book *Jonathan Livingston Seagull*, when, after slamming into a cliff face (symbolizing his death), he awakens in a new and higher dimension (E5).[34]

To try and state this World View in a simpler manner:
1. The creation of the Universe is a neutral transaction;
2. Man's evil nature was introduced for spiritual training (negative transaction);
3. The solution to the problem of evil was supplied by Initiator (positive transaction);
4. Eternity (or the next dimension) is the achievement of the ultimate purpose for each individual life.

Unless and until an individual can adequately resolve all these issues, they are still in the process of maturing. This maturity is not actually and fully achieved by anyone until the E5 has materialized fully.

A brief outline of these 4 foundation elements:
1. The Universe was created at a definable time and operates according to determinable principles. It was established intact and did not come about as the result of a process over immeasurable lengths of time (evolution).

---

[34] *Jonathan Livingston Seagull* by Richard Bach, Pan Books Ltd, 1973

2. Man was introduced into the Creation (a fuller discussion of What Man Is, can be found in our publication *The Greatest Miracle of All*[35]). Into this inherently neutral state, the force of 'evil' was deliberately introduced as part of a training program for the development of character or moral ability. This moral aspect cannot be created. It inherently is a process. Initiator is the Trainer and is accomplishing this program with each individual at a different pace. Completion of (or graduation from) this training only occurs in E5.

3. The negative force has been neutralized by a one-time event of Initiator personally materializing into this dimension (E4), applying and demonstrating this new positive overpowering force, commonly called 'love'. Although this was a one-time event and accomplishment, the negative effects or 'evil' still continue in a controlled manner for training purposes, until the final phase, when it will be totally abolished. The 'evil' or negative force simply has a temporary purpose for training.

4. E4 has a definite end-point, at which time E5 will be introduced. Evil or the negative force and its effects do not exist there. Each and every individual who existed in E4 has a place and purpose in E5.

Response

We have just covered profound concepts, with far-reaching implications on your life. So the question is, what is your reaction to what we have just discussed? You either accepted it as obvious, rejected it outright or have mixed feelings of doubt and possible acceptance. If you are comfortable with the Biblical World View, you may wish to skip ahead to 'Why Did We Prepare This Manual?', the next section on page 112.

Fear, Uncertainty & Doubt

If you are reading this, you understandably have certain reservations about the Biblical World View. That is perfectly acceptable – a healthy dose of skepticism is always called for.

Let us ask a question.

Why could you accept some of the previous illusions we discussed as obvious? Why were you frustrated that we spent so much time discussing them when the illusion was perfectly clear to you? Did you know that some people have extreme difficulty accepting what you have already accepted as obvious?

---

[35] www.freedomtechnology.org/resources/truth/

Similarly, others have felt frustrated that we even discussed the Biblical World View at all – it is perfectly obvious to them.

The reason you could accept certain previous illusions as obvious is because you have seen sufficient evidence to know unequivocally that the illusion we presented was just that: an illusion. The fact that you had seen sufficient evidence was all you needed to identify each illusion.

So, the fact that you doubt the Biblical World View is because you have not yet seen sufficient evidence to convince you.

Or it could be that the contrary evidence you have seen came from a man-made belief system, which we have already accepted is one of the illusions.

Or it could be that Initiator has chosen to not reveal this understanding to you, yet. But it will be revealed to you. Either some time soon while in the E4, or when E5 arrives.

The Test

What you do next is entirely up to you.

You can choose to immediately reject our World View, the empirically proven Biblical World View, in which case the rest of this manual will not interest you in the slightest. Remember that not all people are equal, and we are not going to convince you to change your paradigm, unlike all other religions. We have planted the seed, and that is the only action we have been called on to take.

The other action you can take is to gather the required evidence to support this view.

We will not kid you – the task will not be easy. You are up against the negative force which has a vested interest in disproving the Biblical World View. You will come across mountains of material which appears to be scientifically accurate, and which will disprove the Biblical World View. You will have a challenge sifting fact from fiction. We know, because it is taken us a combined 80-person years to sift through what is available. It is not an easy task.

Or you can choose to blindly accept that our extensive research is sound and can be relied on.

We would not recommend this either. Axiom 1 states that you will not be controlled by anyone, including Freedom Technology. Axiom 11 states that you accept full responsibility for any actions you take. Blindly accepting the Biblical World View is abdicating responsibility to us. This is a form of enslavement, and we do not recommend you do so at all.

What we can recommend is that you apply the test of rationality. Spend the next few days thinking about the Biblical World

View. Does it make sense? Could it provide answers to the confusing state of the world? Does it sound rational?

Re-read this chapter, believing that Initiator will provide you the understanding that has been promised. Perhaps this chapter or even the manual is an aid to understanding. We have also provided numerous Internet links to carefully selected articles on page 237, which will assist in deciding whether the Biblical World View holds water.

You may also want to see our related publications:
- *The Real Truth about Heaven*
- *The Real Truth about Who Will Be Saved: the Few or All*
- For a bird's eye view of the meaning of life, see our publication: *The Greater Picture: Truth, Freedom and Omega Point.*[36]

We wish you clarity and understanding in this most important of life's journeys.

Why Did We Prepare This Manual?

Thus far we believe we have answered all but one of the questions we posed at the beginning of this chapter. The final question is "What is our motive for making this material available?"

Apart from those listed in our Mission Statement, an obvious motive is that we are obligated to explain the Biblical World View. We have introduced it in this chapter, and we will cover more of it in the next section on Metaphysical Truths. But for us the most exciting part about preparing this information is that we believe the significantly challenging process of preparing the manual and finding a publisher who would accept such controversial material, is part of our training for management tasks in the E5.

If that blows you away, you have no idea how excited we are about this concept. Ever woken up in the morning so happy that you have to pinch yourself to see if reality is real? It happens on a daily basis once you have grasped this concept.

There are a few further motives for making this material available, which we will explain now.

Community

Unless you have been wearing blinkers for the past few years, we are entering a tremulous period in time. Things are not as they seem.

Some are referring to this period of time as the End Times. Some are expecting World War Three to occur in the not too distant future. Others are expecting celestial bodies to impact earth, or major tectonic plate movements to cause massive and sustained earthquakes.

We share the general views of the doomsayers, except for the negative connotations. We firmly believe that, although we are entering possibly difficult times, they are also exciting times, and opportunities abound for those who are prepared.

At the end of this manual you will be invited to register your details with a rather unique group – an enlightened community. We currently have no specific plans for this community, although many ideas are being discussed. We have no doubt that a group of like minded contrarian thinkers could achieve spectacular things, and maybe even assist in saving lives when cataclysms start. And we have not even started talking about the Universe Management positions yet – that we will keep for a later chapter. We do not want to blow any fuses now.

Each of us in this community would like to count on the support of other *Fresh Thinkers* when the need arises, as the world slides ever lower into moral and spiritual stagnation.

We hope you feel the same.

Reciprocal Value Exchange

As you have seen, we frequently refer to other publications in the Freedom Technology arsenal of publications. These are information packs unlike anything you will find in bookstores today, and will make the usefulness of anything you have bought previously pale into insignificance.

We believe firmly in all the Axioms, but specifically for this discussion: Axiom 12, which states that "Successful relationships hinge upon a continued and approximately equal exchange of values between the partners. When an imbalance occurs *Fresh Thinkers* either address the imbalance or end the relationship."

We are currently enjoying a relationship, even though we have not yet met in person. You have come to trust the information we are sharing, and we have come to trust that you will not arbitrarily share this information indiscriminately.

We are fully committed to over-delivering in any transaction we may enter into with you in the future. We would like nothing more than to develop a relationship with you, instead of simply providing you with this manual and then leaving you to your own devices.

But this concept becomes even more exciting, because we have a very real and profitable way of generating wealth for you. And it has nothing to do with drawing a salary, selling Multi-Level-Marketing products or any 'money-making scheme' you may have come across in the past.

In the next Wealth Creation section we will reveal to you how this unique method works, and what it means for you. We know you will like the idea.

Now that we have laid all our cards on the table, you are able to make a more informed decision about whether *Fresh Wisdom* and Freedom Technology can offer any value to you. We hope you are as excited as we are about where this could lead.

Can you see how each of the 5 Pillars of Essential Living all of a sudden take on a whole new meaning with our new paradigm of preparing us for management tasks of the Universe?

Relationships: Does your current relationship build on your Universal management skills, or is it holding you back and stifling you?

Health & Longevity: Does your current understanding of health & longevity prepare you for the exciting task of managing the Universe, where time has no meaning? Living to 120 all of a sudden sounds far more interesting than it might have earlier, because there are so many things to prepare ourselves for before we die. What an exciting concept.

Wealth Creation: Does your current understanding of 'value creation' vs. 'value extraction' limit your ability to really make a difference in this dimension, in preparation for the next? Business is not about making money, but about making a positive impact in the lives of those whom you have financial interaction with.

Metaphysical Truths: Can you see how your whole view of religion and spiritual matters takes on a whole new meaning. You will never again be concerned with the pathetic religious arguments most religious people waste their time with.

We will really be cranking up the heat in the second part of each of the 5 Pillars of Fulfilled Living. We think you will agree your patience with the groundwork material is about to be rewarded many times over.

13. Life-Long Love Affairs

Get ready to have your comfort zone stretched and challenged once again.

As a recap, in the first section on Fascinating Relationships we covered the following basics:

-   Most sheep enter into relationships for all the wrong reasons, and end up in a marriage or lifelong relationship which is totally unfulfilling, and becomes a form of entrapment;
-   A fulfilled relationship, on the other hand, commences when both partners believe that the mutual and honest exchange of each other's contribution to the relationship will lead to a temporary increase in happiness for both partners;
-   A fulfilled relationship will end when one or both partners cease to enhance the other's life values; or it will end when one or both partners start to inhibit, destroy or harm the other's life values.

With the basics thus covered, in this section we will be discussing strategies for turning your romantic relationship into a Life-Long Love Affair. We will be covering:

-   **Dating**: the Law of Attraction - Use this Law to find (or keep) your ideal partner and avoid falling for the wrong ones.
-   **Mating**: the Law of Expectations, or what men and women really want out of a relationship.
-   **Ever-Aftering**: the Law of Fidelity between a Woman and a Man that leads to long-term fulfillment, and how to ensure that your relationship becomes a life-long love affair, in which neither partner feels the need to look elsewhere to have their needs fulfilled.

But before we start this discussion, we also need to recap a few important Axioms which we covered earlier and are relevant to this section. The reason will be come clear in a moment.

The Conundrum

If you are in an existing relationship, you may be experiencing a little discomfort right now, as many *Fresh Thinkers* do at this point. Chances are your relationship could very well be violating some of the Axioms we covered previously:

Axiom #1: In order to become free, *Fresh Thinkers* reduce the external controls placed on their life. They will not allow themselves to be controlled by anyone, including a current or future spouse or life partner.

Axiom #4: We recognize that not all people are equal, and will not attempt to convince the sheep of the value of the *Fresh Wisdom*

115

lifestyle. We realize this is an impossible and thankless task. We further realize, whether we like it or not, that this Axiom applies to a spouse we may have married prior to this new understanding.

Axiom #7: The world is, and always has been, an unfair place. *Fresh Thinkers* do not squander their life-energies in an attempt to change this situation. This may include trying to change the belief system of a spouse whom you thought you were 'in love with' but who cannot accept the new understandings you have been learning.

Axiom #8: *Fresh Thinkers* understand that their life has a purpose, even though their purpose may not yet have been fully defined or understood. As far as relationships go, if your spouse does not support your search for your purpose, there is an imbalance in the relationship.

Axiom #11: Responsibility for what happens in the life of a *Fresh Thinker* rests solely with that person. With the new understanding of E4 and E5, a logical extension of this Axiom is that the responsibility given in the next dimension to a *Fresh Thinker* depends entirely on the responsibility shown by that person in the conduct of their life in this dimension.

Axiom #12: Successful relationships hinge upon a continued and approximately equal exchange of values between the partners. When an imbalance occurs *Fresh Thinkers* either address the imbalance or end the relationship.

Hmmm, can you see where this is heading? What does one do if your spouse has no interest in the material we have been covering to date? What does one do if it becomes obvious that your spouse is limiting or even harming your ability to train for management tasks in the E5?

All of a sudden the typical criteria used to define a successful relationship become meaningless.

All of a sudden one has to question whether, in the grander scheme of things, it makes sense to continue with an unfulfilling relationship (no matter how good the sex may be – a common reason for remaining in a relationship).

We are not going to deny that the situation is a tricky one. We know - we have been there before. But as we know by now, we never expect life to be fair.

And we have now reached the stage of *Fresh Wisdom* where we no longer suggest alternatives for you. Remember in the previous chapter we explained that part of our Mission Statement is:

"To open eyes – to stimulate independent thought. We want every *Fresh Thinker* to think for themselves, unlike the sheep who are spoon-fed and hence indoctrinated."

116

So this is a challenge you will have to work through on your own. But we will not leave you completely high and dry. We suggest you work through this entire section on Fascinating Relationships before making any decisions about what to do about your current relationship.

Men and Women

The prime and fundamental Law operating in this area of the 5 Essential Pillars of Fulfilled Living is that men and women are hard-wired. They are pre-programmed. They are built according to a design, a pattern. Men and women are made a certain way, and made to function in different and separate ways. They are designed to complement, or complete, each other. They are two separate halves of an intrinsic whole.

The traditions of today are totally contradictory to the previous paragraph, teaching instead that each person is totally independent of the other. The teachings in this section are based on the Immutable Laws of Nature and are extracted from *Fascinating Womanhood*.[37]

Just as science today can prove beyond any doubt, empirically (that means by evidence), that our Universe was initiated out of nothing, so too it can be demonstrated that we humans have also been 'initiated', created or molded in a certain way.

But, as in so many other aspects of life, distinctions have been lost, polluted, diluted, to the point where there no longer seem to be any absolutes any more.

Pollution of the environment, affecting our whole bodily systems, causing damage to our hormonal balances, among others, has resulted in this specifically male/female aspect of life to become blurred.

Media influence (specifically glossy magazines) is the primary culprit for this blurring of roles.

The roles of the sexes are being confused.

Men are no longer men.

Women are no longer women.

What Fulfilling Relationships require is a return to basic values.

If women are becoming domineering, it may be because men have become weak, spoiled, pampered, spineless for the most part, lacking moral, physical or mental strength or all three.

It is still the fatherless society. The husbands are not husbands. All the women are crying out for a strong man and he is just not there.

---

[37] *Fascinating Womanhood* by Helen Andelin, Bantam Books, 1992.

Many men fail to take their position as head of the household, and allow women and children to push them around, not wishing to accept the responsibility which is rightfully their own.

To a great extent men have failed to assume the responsibility of providing bread for their tables. Women must come to the rescue. Every day millions of women leave their households to assist men in earning the living. The deterioration and loss of effectiveness in so many homes is in great part a consequence of the neglect resulting from the mother deserting her post – a situation she often laments but can do nothing about.

Lack of chivalry (nowadays considered an extremely old-fashioned trait) is apparent on every hand. Women, of necessity, must take care of themselves.

In addition to failing at home, men are failing to measure up in society. We are in a period of crisis where it is likely that the great inheritances we enjoy from the labors and sacrifices of generations past may be lost.

Our only hope is for men to rise to their feet as real men. And for women to support them in this task, by being women.

Where Has the Modern Man Gone Wrong?

The general lack of manliness has produced far-reaching social problems. Men have failed to stand up as the head of the family, and this creates the ongoing strife we see in modern relationships.

There is a lack of order.

The weak-kneed father creates the dominant mother, for someone must add substance to the family life. Someone must determine policy and make decisions. Often urgent demands make it necessary for the wife to step into the leadership role when her husband fails to do so.

Such default in leadership causes great unhappiness and frustration to women. If she must be the man of the family, she is not free to function as a woman, to devote her time and thought to making a success of her equally demanding duties as a wife and mother. Her lack of a strong man to rule over her, something she has every right to expect, may cause severe emotional reactions in her. She tends to become insecure and sometimes desperate.

Children of a recessive father also suffer as innocent victims. They are made to feel insecure due to lack of firmness and decisiveness. Children, who grow up in a home where the father does not command obedience for his word, learn disobedience. They learn that they do not have to yield to authority. When turned out into the world, they become the rebellious youth as we know them today. They are the troublemakers in schools and universities, the lawbreakers and delinquents of society.

The man who allows and encourages his wife to work outside her home creates further social problems. She must divide her interests between her work and family. Since her work is usually more demanding, the children and home life suffer. She cannot serve two masters. Her neglect of home life results in lack of love, attention, and development of the children as well as her failure to serve as the understanding wife.

Abraham Lincoln was described as possessing qualities of steel and velvet. The following is quoted:

"Not often in the story of mankind does a man arrive on earth who is both steel and velvet, who is as hard as a rock and as soft as drifting fog, who holds in his heart and mind the paradox of terrible storm and peace unspeakable and perfect".[38]

Our troubled world requires men of strong minds, kind hearts, and willing hands, men who find joy in labor, men of courage, honor and strong opinions, clear minds and high goals. Men who are not afraid of great responsibility, men who can become dedicated to a task and will surrender their own selfish desires and pursuits to a life of service, men whose word is as good as their bond.

But along with this fiber of steel there must be a gentle nature. We need men who can appreciate a sunrise or a sunset, men who love their families with passion and honor, men who adore womanhood, yet dislike weakness or coyness. We need men with compassion, sensitive to the needs of the less fortunate, men who are tender with their wives and children, men who have developed an ability to love.

The ideal man strives to become a man of Steel and Velvet. It is the way to a man's greatest fulfillment.

Fulfillment does not come, as many suppose, by recognition, honors, money, security, material goods or sexual fulfillment.

Although these attainments contribute greatly to a man's feeling of well-being, his greatest fulfillment comes in being a man.

This goal is attainable, regardless of one's station in life, through the application of definite and unfailing principles.

The Steel

The ideal man has the strength, endurance, and temperance of fine steel.

He is a composite of many sterling qualities. Foremost among them is his willingness to assume masculine burdens, to earn his bread by the sweat of his face, and thus properly provide for himself and

---

[38] As quoted in *Man of Steel and Velvet* by Aubrey Andelin (out of print)

family. He is a man who takes pride in this masculine responsibility. He delights in this opportunity to prove his manhood, and serves with enthusiasm and honor. He does not face his duties sullenly, as though there were no escape, nor does he lean upon society for sustenance. When his problems become difficult, he takes pride in trying to solve them himself. Only in emergencies does he look to others for solutions.

These qualities of masculinity set him apart from women and children and weaker members of his own sex.

A man of steel has a sterling character. He remains steadfast to his convictions even under pressure. He is a man of honor and integrity. He is fair, just and honest in his dealings, possessing moral courage and self dignity and all of those diamond traits which make up a strong character. He becomes master of himself through a conscious effort to incorporate the virtues of strong character in his life. When subjected to pressures, he stands firm.

In addition to all of this, he has achieved a feeling of confidence and peace within which comes from his personal victory over himself. And physically, the man of steel has a body of strength and skill.

The Velvet

The velvet qualities include a man's gentleness, his tenderness, kindness, generosity, and patience. He is devoted to the care and protection of women and children. He understands and respects their gentle nature and recognizes it as a complement to his manliness. He is chivalrous, attentive and respectful to the gentler sex and has an ability to love with tenderness. He has, in addition, an enthusiastic and youthful attitude of optimism which defies the press of years. Humility is also a part of the velvet, subduing the masculine ego as his rough nature is refined.

When properly blended, these traits of steel and velvet compose the ideal man, a masterpiece of creation and the greatest contribution to the well-being of society.

Where Has the Modern Woman Gone Wrong?

Glossy magazines and much of the rest of the media portray the ideal modern woman as someone who:
- is independent
- is aggressive
- earns her own money
- is a sexual hunter/predator
- is domineering, wears the pants in her relationship
- is demanding in what she wants from men

- tries to change her man to comply with what she wants him to do or to be
- has a career outside the home.

Under the guise of *equality, feminism, woman's lib* etc., values like these have been promoted in the media for at least the last 50 years. Without getting into debates about the pros and cons of each movement, what equality of the sexes really means, is freedom for women. It is obvious that this change of values has had a direct impact on society. Here are just a few examples:

- Women tend to transfer their natural respect (and often affection, due to the amount of time spent with him) for their husbands onto their boss. How often does this not lead to affairs - often breaking up not one, but two families?
- Children come home from school to an empty house and grow up in front of the TV, absorbing the values promoted by the mass media; or to child minders who do not have the bandwidth or inclination to address the child's needs.
- Women develop an independent, competitive "I do not need you" attitude toward their partner, instead of one of mutual respect and caring.
- Men become confused as their traditional roles are undermined. They lose self-esteem as they see themselves as no longer being able to support the family, or make decisions for the family.
- Men become miserable and rebellious as they are forced to change into doing things or becoming someone they do not want to. This rebelliousness can easily lead to unintentional straying or affairs.
- Men lose their tenderness and affection for their partner, as instead of someone to cherish and care for, she has become a competitor both in the workplace and at home.

A Solution

Contrast this picture with a feminine woman who has a sense of quiet, inner happiness and contentment about her, a woman who understands men and treats them with respect and admiration, a woman who radiates health and joy as opposed to being obsessed with her looks and figure, plastering herself with makeup in order to feel attractive. Picture too a woman with a sense of self-worth and a good character, one who treats all people well, especially those close to her, because she has a natural respect for all humankind.

This woman can also be playful, fun, charming and childlike when she wants to. A woman like this is truly fascinating to a man. Her good character arouses feelings near worship in a man. Her human

121

qualities fascinate, amuse, enchant and arouse a tender desire to protect her in a man.

This is what an ideal woman looks like. It is the way to a woman's greatest fulfillment and happiness.

What is a Woman's Greatest Need?

Is it to have a lovely home? Happy and healthy children? A successful husband? Time for talents? No financial concerns? Husband and wife having fun together? Is it the feeling of being a successful homemaker? Is it to be admired by her associates? A successful husband who provides economic security?

All of these things are important and some essential, but one need is fundamental.

She must feel loved and cherished by her husband. Without his love, her life is an empty shell.

In accomplishing this, the ideal woman loses none of her dignity, influence, or freedom, but gains them, and it is only then that she can play her vital part in this world. The role of a woman, when played correctly, is fulfilling, fascinating, and full of intrigue. There never need be a dull moment. The practice of this art of womanhood is an enjoyable one, filled with rich rewards, numerous surprises, and vast happiness.[39]

Marriage

For many, the preceding description of the ideal man and woman is simply too old fashioned to contemplate. Hence the sad state of modern relationships.

Those who do understand the value in becoming a person as described will immediately recognize the challenge of finding a spouse who meets this demanding list of ideals. Most people have been brainwashed beyond being useful, and so the question of marriage arises, and the search for the ideal spouse.

The first question to ask is "What needs do you wish to meet in a marriage?"

The male *Fresh Thinker* realizes that he wants women for many different things. The female *Fresh Thinker* realizes that she wants men for many different things. We do not confuse these things in our mind, and attempt to lump them all under one heading called 'love'.

This knowledge confers great power on *Fresh Thinkers*. It enables them to focus their energies on their true desires. It prevents

---

[39] Extracted and adapted from *Fascinating Womanhood* by Helen Andelin, Bantam Books, 1992. First published 1965.
See http://fascinatingwomanhood.net/books/bookshlf.html

them from marrying or living with a partner who they just want to have sex with.

It prevents them from wasting years of their lives with partners who only fill a tiny range of their needs.

It allows them to recognize the many grades and types of 'love', and take rational and logical decisions concerning each one of them.

This knowledge prevents one from marrying for spiritual love, and expecting a super-raunchy sex-life with the same partner. These are not mutually exclusive, of course, just highly unlikely.

This knowledge prevents you from trying to bed your close friends and associates, when this could result in the loss of more valuable aspects of these relationships.

Here are just a few of the things which men and women want from each other (we are not necessarily referring to marriage – simply any relationship between the sexes):

- Spiritual or 'true' love (as distinguished from sexual infatuation);
- Companionship to avoid loneliness;
- Sex with no strings attached;
- Friendship;
- Someone to care for;
- Someone who will take care of them;
- Someone to boost their ego and make them feel good;
- A house-keeper, servant, man-about-the-house, or mechanic;
- An attractive escort;
- A father or mother for their children;
- A husband or wife because peers are pressuring them into marriage;
- Someone to dominate;
- Someone to dominate them;
- A life partner to share their hopes, fears, values, beliefs and ambitions.

Quite a substantial list of needs, is it not?

Yet the average person does not even realize that they require most of these needs to be met in their life. Instead, they are happy to go 'doe-eyed' and 'fall in love' and marry a person who fills one, or perhaps two of the above list. In many cases, a man will 'fall in love' because he wants sex - and be totally unaware (as the sheep nearly always are) of exactly what he is allowing to happen to him.

Fresh Thinkers recognize that they have many different needs concerning relationships. They do not expect to find all of these things in one partner. In fact, they would be amazed and startled if they were to discover a person who filled more than three or four of these needs.

The result is this:

Male *Fresh Thinkers* have many different women to fulfill different needs. He might choose one or more women for sex, a different woman for intellectual discussions, a different woman again to be the mother of his children, and so on. Of course there will be much overlap between these women, and ideally it would be perfect if he could find one woman to fill most of his needs, but he knows that he lives in a real world, with real people, and he knows that statistically it is most unlikely that he will find one woman to fill half of his needs, let alone all of them.

Female *Fresh Thinkers* have many different men to fulfill different needs. She might choose one or more men for sex, a different man for intellectual discussions, a different man again to be the father of her children, and so on. Of course there will be much overlap between these men, and ideally it would be perfect if she could find one man to fill most of her needs, but she knows that she lives in a real world, with real people, and she knows that statistically it is most unlikely that she will find one man to fill half of her needs, let alone all of them.

Remember, we are talking about *Fresh Thinkers* here, not sheep. If a *Fresh Thinker* desires a house-keeper or servant, then they will employ one, not marry one. If they desire great sex with many different partners, then they will seek this out, and not marry the first person who agrees to go to bed with them. If a woman desires a charming, handsome escort then she will have an array of men who are willing to fill this desire. She will not marry the first sweet-talking bozo she stumbles across.

Life Sentence

The sheep allow biological programming to rule their lives. They are more or less incapable of discerning what is really happening when they 'fall in love', with the result that they make costly mistakes. These mistakes can, and do, remove ten or twenty years from their lives. But this is considered normal by the sheep, and so they rarely question it.

'Normal' men marry (for example) beautiful, curvy, sexy blondes when they really might only want sex with these women. Their ideal partner might be quiet, loving, supportive and kind.

'Normal' women marry (for example) handsome, smooth-talking, charming hunks, when their ideal partner might be caring, supportive, kind, loving, capable, dependable etc.

As we have said many times, the sheep rarely know their true motives for doing anything (axiom #8). This certainly includes 'falling in love' and 'getting married' (or equivalent).

We know that this is a somewhat stark view of relationships. Our intention is to make some general points about the real nature of 'romantic love' as practiced by the majority of sheep. We want to smash the illusion so that you, as an aspiring *Fresh Thinker*, can be free of this crazy myth. A *Fresh Thinker* is able to love openly, honestly, and in a non-controlling manner.

We refuse to play any mind games. Instead, we openly and honestly tell our partner what we desire from them. If they decide to give it, fantastic, otherwise the *Fresh Thinker* will seek other partners who will provide for their needs.

Please re-read the above paragraph, because it has profound implications for how you should conduct your romantic/sex-life from now on, if you aspire to become a *Fresh Thinker*.

This is not a purely 'taking' process, of course. Your relationships should be similar to a fair and reasonable business trade. Few prospective partners will give without receiving roughly equal value in return (unless they are conned by a sheep using one or more of the common illusions and tricks).

The point here is that the sheep are always trying to con each other (because they are largely unfamiliar with indulging in 'straight' transactions). Here's how it works:

1. Women attempt to con men into marrying them (or a long-term relationship). They use many weapons to do this, often subconsciously. They will promise a man that which he most desires (sex or acknowledgement) in return for that which she most desires (security). They often have no intention of delivering for longer than it takes to trap the man. This duplicity is often subconscious on their part; they might even claim to be 'in love' with the man.

2. Men attempt to con women into having sex with them. They use all of the weapons to do this, but typically they will promise a woman that which she most desires (security), in return for sex. They often have no intention of delivering for longer than it takes to bed the woman.

Women are often <u>not</u> fully aware that they are conning the man. Men are often fully aware that they are conning the woman.

Yes, we know, all men and women are not like this. We are generalizing to make a point.

Tough Questions to Ask About Marriage

In this section we will purely pose a few questions and leave you to answer them for yourself. The extent to which you genuinely question these firmly held beliefs is the extent to which you will be able to free yourself from a potentially limiting relationship. As a start to answering the questions, you might want to see *The History of Love and Sex.*[40]

1. During what periods in history was it accepted for men to have more than one wife?
2. What were the reasons given for the increased success of unions between multiple women and a man?
3. When (how recently) was the concept of a monogamous marriage introduced?
4. What are the reasons given for the high modern divorce rate?
5. What does the Bible (not your mythical religious fables and traditions) teach about sex and marriage?

Once you have considered the implications of modern marriage, you will realize that it is a manufactured con, designed to enslave non-thinking sheep in a lifetime of misery.

That does not mean marriage and log-term relationships cannot work. Rather, the basis on which these relationships are formed need to be readdressed.

As an alternative, we have provided suggested open, honest and frank marriage vows in Appendix B – Suggested Wedding Vows on page 230. You can also find an interesting *Contract for Unmarried Cohabitation or Marriage* online[41].

At this point, we must stress that we are not on a crusade to abolish marriage or attempt to get everyone to start enjoying honest, open and genuine relationships with each other. We merely wish to point out that most people plunge into boring, sterile, hurtful and dishonest relationships with each other - and stick it out until they die. We hope by now you know enough to be guilt-free in this matter.

Dating

Have you ever noticed that women do not seem to make sense at all when it comes to dating? You have probably been in a situation where you really liked a woman, and you did everything right... but for some reason she just never felt attracted to you.

You called her often, took her to nice places, bought her gifts, and were a complete gentleman, but nothing seemed to cause her to like you for more than just a friend.

What is going on here?

In dating there is a Fundamental Law of Attraction, which has become totally blurred and unrecognizable by the media who are intent on selling you products which improve only the exterior. Any man or woman who understands this Law can use it to get whatever or whomever they want.

[40] www.neo-tech.com/history/
[41] www.neo-tech.com/love-contract/

Therefore it is absolutely necessary for men and women to understand this Law, both to identify and then to become attached to the ideal partner.

The Fundamental Law of Attraction

Men are pre-wired to want to be appreciated, accepted and admired above all else.

Knowing this, an unscrupulous woman can win any man away from his partner merely by giving him this. Not sex. Just look at the kind of women who lure men away. Completely irrational – so it seems.

Women are pre-wired to want a dominant male.

But, as discussed earlier, such men are few and far between.

So, any man who can learn what it is that women respond to, such as confidence and playfulness; arrogance tinged with humor - can captivate any woman, regardless of the way he looks, since women are not so much attracted by appearance as men are.

Men are more attracted to physical traits and women are more attracted to personality traits.

Men are sexually aroused and turned on instantly at the sight of a young, shapely female body. As a man, you know that this process happens instantly and 'all by itself', meaning you do not really have a choice in the matter.

The same is true for women, who are sexually aroused initially and turned on when they interact with a man that has certain qualities and personality traits.

Women become instantly turned on sexually when they are in the presence of certain personality traits, just like men become turned on by certain physical traits. Think about that for a moment.

Men become turned on by what they can see. Women become turned on by what can never be seen.

And even when it comes to the physical, women are still more interested in the *how* than the *what*.

It is not as much his body as the way a man holds it and carries it. It is not as much his voice as the way a man uses it.

Do physical looks, money, fame, power, height, age, etc. play into this at all?

Of course they do. But they are not nearly as important as most men think they are.

If you are tall, handsome, rich, and famous... great. You will probably have an easier time attracting women. This can open the door for a guy, but it does not at all guarantee that the woman will stay around. There are many rich, famous, powerful men who still have no success with women.

To sum up: Attraction is different for men than it is for women.

While men are attracted mostly by physical traits, women are attracted mostly by personality traits.

Women do not decide who to feel attracted to with their logical minds. They decide with their emotions, and then make up reasons and rationalize it.

Attraction is not a choice!

This is why some men attract women so well, while others do not... and why any man can improve his success with women dramatically, no matter what his looks, age, or income.

Please think about what you have just read, and pay attention when you are out watching men and women interact.

Start noticing those things that men are doing to attract women that are related to their personalities and their communication with women. You will see things you have never seen before, and learn secrets that will improve your success with women tremendously.

If you want to learn more about the Law of Attraction for Men, we recommend *Double Your Dating*.[42]

Mating

The principles of mating, or sexual union, are based on the scientifically absolute realities that all advanced scientists, including Einstein and Stephen Hawking, agree:

Our world did not evolve, but was created by an Initiator outside of this system. Not only that, but scientific evidence indicates that this Initiator created a Universe that is exquisitely fine-tuned for the support of physical life and especially for the support of human beings. In fact, the Universe is designed specifically to make the existence of humans possible[43].

When we understand all the above, we know that we sexual beings are also made in a certain way and we function best when we know and understand the basics of how this most exciting aspect of existence, the relationship between the sexes, works.

We are going to be talking openly and frankly about sex, because some basics will go a long way towards making the emergence into a sexual relationship more harmonious and longer lasting. Instead of assuming that we just have to find the right person who will 'make us satisfied' and having a string of relationships in this hope, why not look to improving our own performance in this area, making it possible to have longer lasting relationships. We are going to look at sex from a biological and scientific perspective. You may be shocked, but

---

[42] www.FreedomTechnology.org/resources/relationships.htm
[43] *A Brief History of Time* by Stephen W. Hawking, Bantam Press 1988

hopefully by now we no longer need to make excuses for the frank manner we expose the cons we have been subject to.

It is reality the way it really is.

What is Sex Really?

Sex has been shrouded in mystery. What is it? Is it sacred or is it sin? Should we do it or should we not? Who should we do it with? Should we do it with just one person? Why do we enjoy it? How can we enjoy it more? How is sex related to love? Is it wrong or is it right? How can something so necessary be wrong? How can something so undignified be so right?

Animals do not have these problems with sex because they do not have the ability to ask questions. Animals just have sex. They have no choice. It is instinct. It is what they do. It is what they have been doing for the last thirty thousand years. The animals that did not have sex failed to reproduce and became extinct. A species' ability to survive depended on its ability to reproduce.

But what about people? We are not mere animals are we? Are we not somehow higher than the animals? Are we not somehow above mere reproduction? Surely there are some differences between us and the beasts are there not?

To best understand sex we have to put aside our mythical and religious views and get down to the fundamentals. Once we know what sex is and why we do it, we can better understand how to do it right. We are now going to have that little talk about 'the birds and the bees' in a way you might not have heard it before.

The closer you get to the biological reproductive instincts that we all have, the hotter the sex is.

The primary reason for sex is having babies. That is what sex is for. So yes, we are like the animals. And when it comes to sex we are more like the animals than anything else we do is. Sex is not optional. We have sex because we have to. It is instinct. We are beasts in a world of beasts and we have sex because our parents and all our ancestors did. And we will have children and they will have sex and have children. And that is the basis of what sex is all about.

We are male and female. Our bodies are designed for sex. A woman has a vagina for a single reason: to receive a penis and cause him to ejaculate in her so she will receive his genetic material, become pregnant, and have a baby. Our bodies are designed to accomplish this and that is the biological goal behind sex.

You might now be thinking, 'I do not have sex because I want babies. I have sex for fun.' Yes, that is true. In fact sex is so much fun that you cannot help but to have it. If sex were not so much fun we would not be doing it and if we did not do it, humans would not be around very long. Sex is fun because if sex were not fun, we would not be here.

Fresh Thinkers believe that romantic love has, as its primary drive, the purely biological function of sexual reproduction. In other words, lurking just below the surface of romantic love is the not so romantic desire to reproduce.

We are all biologically programmed to reproduce. This is our primary directive, because without this, all other directives (to eat, to survive) are pointless.

If you were writing a program to control human beings in order to ensure that they reproduced as often as possible, you would probably include the following elements:

-   Ensure that both men and women are fairly obsessed with sex (they are);
-   Ensure that women feel more romantic and sexy during ovulation (they do);
-   Invent an overwhelming emotion which overrides all logic, rational thought and common sense and ensures that male and female couple together, no matter what. We call this 'being in love';
-   On the basis of maximizing reproduction, ensure that men want to have sex with as many different women as possible (they do);
-   Ensure that the man has an orgasm a long time before the woman, otherwise the woman would have her orgasm, push the man off before he has his, and thereby prevent conception.

Is it just a staggering coincidence that the program which controls our sexual and romantic feelings, happens to be exactly the one which also maximizes the chance of reproduction?

For more information on Advanced Sexual Techniques, see our publication *How To Do Great Sex - It is Easier Than You Think.*[44]

Space and time restrict us from going into a long discussion of why we have been lied to so that we believe what we currently do about sex. We have been manipulated by religion and health scares about enjoying sex the way it was meant to be enjoyed. Very often sex is mistakenly used as the reason relationships break down, and yet nothing could be further from the truth.

The main reason relationships break down is because the primary need of man is not met in most relationships: *the need to be appreciated, admired and respected.*

---

[44] www.freedomtechnology.org/resources/sex

The main reason relationships break down is because the primary need of woman is not met in most relationships: *the need to be cherished and adored.*

For Ever Aftering

After much negative discussion on relationships (which was necessary to break any previous held limiting beliefs) we at last come to the part of Fascinating Relationships that shows how to have a life-long love affair with your partner.

Do not get us wrong: we do not regard the State sponsored marriage license that the State requires as the only answer. In earlier times a marriage was when 2 people came before their community and friends and announced publicly their intention to live together. It was a social, not a civil undertaking.

Subsequently the State has jumped in and formalized this relationship too, taking even greater control in individuals' lives.[45] As the *Fresh Thinker* knows, we wish to avoid any unnecessary controls in our lives, including that of the State.

The fundamental Universal Principles in the area of life-long fulfilling relationships are:

1. She must feel loved and cherished by her husband. A man's most important responsibility in life is to be the guide, protector and provider for his wife and children. This role is not merely a result of custom or tradition, but is of divine origin.
2. He must feel appreciated and accepted for who he is. A man wants a woman who will place him at the top of her priority list, not second but first. He wants to be the king-pin around which all other activities of her life revolve. Children miss nothing when their father comes first, but rather feel more secure and happy.

When a Man Fails In His Role

A failure in the home is a man's greatest failure. If he fails in marriage, if he fails with his children, if his home is troubled or divided by divorce, or if his children are unruly, wayward or irresponsible, he has failed in his most fundamental duties as a man. No success in life can compensate for this failure in the home. A failure in the home has direct implications on the amount of responsibility given in the E5.

The home is the most basic unit of society. The strength of a country lies in the home and the security and happiness of the family. It

---

[45] www.wealth4freedom.com/truth/mpl_birthcertificate.shtml - Did the State Pledge Your Body to a Bank?

is difficult, if not impossible, for the man, the woman or the children to give much of value to the world if their home is troubled.

When a Man Succeeds In His Role

On the positive side, when a man functions well as the guide, protector and provider, when his home is ruled with firmness and kindness, love and good leadership, with the security and comforts that are necessary, and when his children develop into happy, well-adjusted citizens, then has he made his most notable contribution to his society and the world.

It has been said that one sign of a man's success is demonstrated when he walks up the path leading to his home and his children run with eagerness to greet him, and his wife, smiling, lovingly greets him at the door This is a man's greatest success and therefore his greatest achievement.

The most important way a man can contribute to the security and happiness of his marriage is to successfully live his masculine role. This means, in review, that he rules his household with firmness, kindness, and love . . . that he provides an adequate living, that he protects his wife and children and in every way serves as a man. In addition, if he will learn to understand women and children, and contribute to their needs, he will achieve a happy marriage.

What the Modern Woman Does not Realize

Possibly the largest con imposed on women today is the desire to be equal with men, when the Universal Law is to make him number one.

What the modern woman does not realize is that it is not a desire for sex that drives unfaithful partners to other women. It is not sex he needs from other women but acceptance, admiration, and being number one. If the woman treats him like a king, he will treat her like a queen.

When a woman lives these concepts devotedly, her partner will be tender and romantic. She will be not only loved, but cherished, honored, and adored. These principles make women happier, men happier, and children happier. One woman said, "Even my dog is happier."[46]

A woman is in a precarious position as the wife. She can build or destroy him. She destroys him by needling him to change, stealing his leadership, wounding his pride, and ignoring his important needs. She builds him up by appreciating him, and admiring him.

---

[46] Quoted in *Fascinating Womanhood* by Helen Andelin, Bantam Books, 1992.

The Complementary Partnership

The greatest success in a relationship occurs when husband and wife devotedly live their respective roles. In the ideal home the man's and woman's duties are distinctly divided. There is little overlapping except in emergencies.

It is a fundamental fact that men and women differ temperamentally, psychologically, physically, socially and in capacity to do a specific job. Although they are equal in intelligence, their intelligence is not on identical subjects. They do not think alike, have the same perspectives, nor do they react in the same way to a given circumstance. They worry about different things, and they worry differently. Men and women do not have the same capacity in a specific job.

We fully realize that this concept goes against the grain of every modern teaching on relationships. Women are taught to strive for 'equality with men'. The media's greatest success has been in the area of relationships, marriage and love.

Obviously many people will do whatever they are told and imitate whatever is presented as 'current trends'. They have not yet learned to distrust the media, government and education, so the principles expounded in soap operas and in glossy magazines are lapped up with glee.

Female empowerment is a cruel hoax. It flatters and lures young women with money and recognition and paints marriage and family in a dreary light. Thus many women are deprived of a lifetime of love from husband and children.

If you are interested in reading further how this simple principle has been used effectively to destroy the family unit, we encourage you to read an article online with an open and enquiring mind (including all the links referenced and positive and negative comments from readers): *The Hoax of Female Empowerment*[47].

Is Your Relationship a Ten?

Building and maintaining a great relationship with your special someone is an all-the-time endeavor.

The following simple process is one you can use for any relationship – personal, professional, co-worker, boss, friend or business partner.

If we really care about a relationship, we have to regularly check on how we are doing. We cannot depend upon the other party to always tell us what is working and what is not.

---

[47] www.savethemales.ca/001170.html

Here is the sequence: Ask them, "On a scale of one to ten, how would you rate our relationship?" And then wait for the answer.

If they are slow to respond, you may want to jump into the silence. Resist that temptation.

If they rate your relationship anything less than ten, ask, "What would it take to make it a ten?" Again, it is worth the wait for answers that will give you important insight into what the other person wants and needs.

Assumptions can wound or even kill the best of relationships.

These simple questions can keep assumptions from hurting your relationship and help you develop a deeper, more fulfilling one.

It may seem uncomfortable at first, but it becomes easier and more effective the more the exercise is repeated over time. It is often a conversation that will continue over several sessions.

It is a great springboard for some in-depth discussions, so get ready for some breakthroughs.

7 Common Relationship Mistakes

Keep your relationship out of danger by avoiding the 7 common mistakes that can lead to failure.

Getting your relationship to last may actually be more of a science than you think. When numerous relationship experts were consulted for a recent study, there was a general consensus that the following seven factors were key to determining whether a relationship would succeed or fail:

1. Couples who are too closely entwined are often the most fragile. They live as one until one day something comes along and pushes them apart – a child, a new-found interest for one of the partners, or simply one of the partners suddenly becomes overcome by a feeling of boredom or suffocation;
2. Failure to accept that the other partner is very different – notably because they are of a different sex – and does not always see things in the same way as you;
3. Lack of communication – especially when a couple feels that the instinct of love should be enough of a communication to bond them in itself and does not make a big effort to communicate about what is going on, or going wrong;
4. Situations where one of the partners takes on the role of 'looking after' the other – whether they have emotional problems, life problems or addictions to drugs or alcohol;
5. Where one or both of the partners lacks a personal 'life project' – something that absorbs them, excites them and gives their life meaning;

6. Laziness and complacency – because as with all things you want to do well in life, you have to work at it;
7. Giving in – to the loss of the sexual side of the relationship, and to conflicts that you no longer bother trying to work through because you think it is too late.

~~~

We only regard those unions as real examples of love and real marriages in which a fixed and unalterable decision has been taken. If men or women contemplate an escape, they do not collect all their powers for the task. In none of the serious and important tasks of life do we arrange such a "getaway." We cannot love and be limited. – Alfred Adler

Love at first sight is easy to understand; it's when two people have been looking at each other for a lifetime that it becomes a miracle. – Amy Bloom

There are two dilemmas that rattle the human skull: How do you hang on to someone who won't stay? And how do you get rid of someone who won't go? – Danny deVito, *The War of the Roses*

Some people claim that marriage interferes with romance. There's no doubt about it. Anytime you have a romance, your wife is bound to interfere. – Groucho Marx

There is nothing nobler or more admirable than when two people who see eye to eye keep house as man and wife, confounding their enemies and delighting their friends. - Homer

What you are as a single person, you will be as a married person, only to a greater degree. Any negative character trait will be intensified in a marriage relationship, because you will feel free to let your guard down -- that person has committed himself to you and you no longer have to worry about scaring him off. – Josh McDowell

The sharing of joy, whether physical, emotional, psychic, or intellectual, forms a bridge between the sharers which can be the basis for understanding much of what is not shared between them, and lessens the threat of their difference. – Audre Lorde

14. The Age Conspiracy

There are literally thousands of alternative health regimes available today, some good, others created by giant pharmaceutical firms and simply branded 'Alternative'.

Very few health strategies focus on longevity. Because of society's obsession with quick fixes, many alternative health strategies provide rapid solutions, but in doing so tend to damage your long-term health. The authors have spent many years researching emerging strategies that indicate that being active and well to 120 is a reasonable goal. Many researchers are now pushing the 130 and 140 year barrier. Some are even talking about reversing aging completely.[48]

It is often assumed that the average human lifespan is 70 years (three score and ten, as quoted in the Bible). This is false for two reasons: Biblically, and Scientifically.

The Real Biblical Age Story

Prior to the Biblical Flood, men and women used to live to many hundreds of years, with Methuselah reaching 969, Jared 962, and Mahalel 895.

But mankind rebelled and chose to ignore the Immutable Laws of Nature (or the laws laid down by God). God decided to end the wickedness by sending a flood. At the same time He decided to curtail their lifespan.

Then the Lord said, My spirit shall not for ever dwell and strive with man, for he also is flesh; but his days shall be 120 years.[49]
After the flood Noah lived another 350 years, dying at age 950, while others lived substantially shorter periods after the flood: Shem, 600; Arpachshad, 438; Shelah 433; Reu, 239; Nahor, 148[50].

Abraham lived to 175[51] and Sarah to 127[52].

Now we need to deal with the so-called 'three score and ten' lifespan.

This expression in Psalm 90 has been taken out of context and misapplied. Psalm 90 is in essence a plea by Moses to re-consider the curse of 40 years imposed on the faithless Israelites.

Quoting from the Amplified Version: "For we [the Israelites in the wilderness] are consumed by your anger, and by your wrath we are troubled, overwhelmed and frightened away... For all our days [out here in this wilderness, says Moses] are passed away in Your wrath; we

---

[48] www.gen.cam.ac.uk/sens/
[49] Genesis 6:3
[50] Genesis 11
[51] Genesis 25:7
[52] Genesis 23:1

spend our years as a tale that is told [for we adults know we are doomed to die soon, without reaching Canaan]... Who knows the power of your anger? [Who worthily connects this brevity of life with your recognition of sin?] And your wrath, who connects it with the reverent and worshipful fear that is due to You? So, teach us to number our days that we may get us a heart of wisdom."[53]

[Note from the authors: remember why God brought about the Flood mentioned earlier].

Psalm 90v13 - Turn, O Lord [from Your fierce anger]; {for how long?} Revoke Your sentence and be comforted and eased towards Your servants.

Within *this* context we read verse 10:

Psalm 90v10 - The days of our years are three score and ten.

The note in the Amplified version to this verse reads: *"This Psalm is credited to Moses, who is interceding with God to remove the curse which made it necessary for every Israelite over the age of 20 (when they rebelled at Kadesh-Barnea) to die before reaching the Promised Land."*

Moses says most of them are dying at age 70. This number has often been mistaken as a set span of life for mankind. It was not intended to refer to any one except to those Israelites under the curse during that particular forty years. Seventy years has never been the average span of life for humanity. When Jacob, the father of the 12 tribes had reached 130 years[54], he complained that he had not attained to the years of his immediate ancestors. In fact Moses himself lived to be 120, Aaron 123, Miriam several years older, and Joshua 110; David 140; while in the Millennium a person dying at 100 will still be a child.[55]

Also, traditionally the age of *majority* or *manhood* was 30. After which a man could usually marry, transact etc. This is probably the reason Moses says '70' in verse 10, being 30 plus the 40 years of the curse.

And so it appears obvious that the '70 years' of Psalm 90v10 is not to be taken as the expected lifespan upon a Biblical basis.

The Scientific Reality of Age

Any Biologist will tell you that human cells seem to have a built-in time clock: they keep renewing themselves until approximately age 120, when the Biological Clock seems to run down and the cells stop reproducing.

[53] Psalm 90:7-12
[54] Genesis 47:9
[55] Isaiah 65:20

By 2050, "the number of US centenarians is expected to reach 834,000 and maybe even 1 million," said Dr. Robert Butler, President of the International Longevity Center in New York City.[56]

Leading-edge technology is currently looking at ways to push that barrier to 130 and 140, simply accepting that the present barrier is only 120.

The average lifespan of medical doctors in the USA is currently 6.7 years *shorter* than the average for the population as a whole.[57] Which leads one to surmise that part of the problem may well lie with the advice being dispensed (albeit unintentionally) by the Medical Industry.

Dr Walford (one of the leading exponents of living to 120 - having published major works, *The 120 Year Diet* and *Beyond The 120-Year Diet* [58]) has determined that one of the most promising ways of extending life (and this is the new concept – Life Extension, as opposed to simply health) is the Hi - Low diet: High Nutrient Density and Low Volume.

In other words, no junk food that contains calories devoid of nutrition, and a focus on foods with high nutrient values.

The underlying basis is that the stomach and how it is treated affects the lifespan.

Another technology that is prominent (there are more of this particular type of practitioners in Hollywood than anywhere else on earth) is Chelation, the intravenous application of a substance called EDTA. We introduced this therapy in an earlier chapter.

Chelation is simply the eradication of free radicals and metals (especially heavy metals) from the system.

Chelation practitioners simply say the following: "Not one of our patients ever dies of cancer!"

That is how powerful this therapy is.

These are the most important strategies that anyone seeking to extend their length of life, can apply, as at this writing. Let us look into Chelation a little more.

A Consumer's Guide to Chelation Therapy

The following section is summarized from the fantastic book on Chelation Therapy called *Forty-Something Forever.*[59]

Since this section is merely a summary of their detailed book, we have left out all names, footnotes and references, but they are all included in their book, which is extremely well researched and

---

[56] http://en.wikipedia.org/wiki/Centenarian
[57] http://skepdic.com/deaddocs.html
[58] *Beyond The 120 Year Diet* by Roy L. Walford M.D. www.walford.com/120diet.htm
[59] *Forty-Something Forever* by Harold and Arlene Brecher, Health Savers Press, 1992

documented. We encourage you to track down a copy (they can be rather elusive because of the suppression this therapy suffers from).

If you are over 40 and concerned about longevity, or have symptoms of any of the diseases mentioned on page 56, the Brecher's book is a must-read.

Introduction

Chelation therapy is a process involving the use of chelating agents[60] such as EDTA[61] to remove heavy metals, free radicals and other toxins from the body.

The chelating agent may be administered intravenously, intramuscularly, or orally, depending on the agent and the type of poisoning.

With the twin fields of Free Radical Pathology and Bio-Oxidative Medicine, we can make living to 120 a reasonable goal, and in so doing, indefinitely extend 'middlescence'.

Dr. Elmer M. Cranton, M.D. describes Chelation in his book, *Bypassing Bypass Surgery*[62], as "a non-surgical treatment for reversing arteriosclerosis, improving blocked circulation, and slowing the aging process".

A Hospital Is Not A Place To Get Well

In a recent Harvard study it was found that just over 50% of US hospitals did not properly monitor patients. Harvard concluded that negligence kills thousands each year and injures many more.[63] There are frequent failures of technology exacerbated by the employment of untrained technicians to keep costs down. 10,000 deaths per year are attributable to anesthesia, and Harvard suspects it could be 3 to 4 times higher. Common errors are syringe swapping, ampoule swapping, drug overdoses, and incorrect drugs administered. 2 million or more get sicker instead of better. There are 100,000 hospital-originated, infection-related deaths each year. Harvard says it is super-conservative to claim that at least 20% of in-patients leave with a condition they did not have on entering.

Prescription medication is the sixth leading cause of death in the USA, according to the Center for Disease Control.[64]

---

[60] http://en.wikipedia.org/wiki/Chelation
[61] http://en.wikipedia.org/wiki/EDTA
[62] http://drcranton.com/bypass.htm
[63] http://nwhalliance.org/harvard.htm
[64] www.cdc.gov/nchs/fastats/lcod.htm

Chelation Suppressed

250,000 heart bypass operations are performed each year in the US. A careful look at the results reveals it does not help the vast majority.

"It is a crime," charges Dr. E. W. McDonagh who has assembled thousands of documented cases histories of recovered 'untreatable' patients, "that news of this breakthrough treatment for heart, diabetes, stroke and other diseases has been purposely withheld from the public" (referring to Chelation).[65]

Most medical white papers routinely refuse all pro-Chelation stories.

How blatantly corrupt have the anti-Chelation forces been? They have resorted to massive pro-bypass propaganda to blast the Chelation alternative out of the picture.

Why Is The Medical Industry Against Chelation?

Medical politics and Chelation threatens the financial well-being of a politically powerful and well established branch of the medical profession.

The average citizen, not privy to behind-the-scenes shenanigans of pharmaceutical, medical and food industry cronies, would be shocked to learn to what extent these powerhouses are able to distort science news.

Too many health professionals have too much to gain from the bypass industry to call a halt. Anesthetists, operating team personnel, coronary care unit staff, radiologists, technicians, hospital administrators - some forty-five specialists in all.

The Brecher's provide well-researched lists of referenced proofs that Chelation is either purposely shunned, or even forcefully suppressed.

Sixty Minutes is not interested in covering Chelation; neither is The Washington Post, The Larry King Show, or Phil Donahue.

Chelation therapy is potentially so costly to the insurance industry they cannot afford to have it approved (meaning that premiums will be reduced because of the reduced cost of treatment).

The large medical centers are co-conspirators. High-tech in-hospital procedures have grown to a $6billion annual bonanza. Chances are you will call Chelation a bargain. You will cut future drug and medical bills and enjoy added years of pleasurable and productive activity. What a deal!

Surgeons get paid top dollar - $383,520 p/a. Other medical specialists get $250,000 to $300,000, and that is without including the kickbacks from pacemaker manufacturers, referral dividends from

---

[65] www.bonniecolton.com/1997.htm

investments in multi-million dollar CAT scan and MRI imaging centers and profits from doctor-owned pharmacies.

When doctors face life or death decisions themselves, they shun their own advice and turn to Chelation. Thousands are secretly Chelated every year.[66]

A Miracle Cure-All?

We will let Chelated patients tell you in their own words:

"Your treatments have turned my life around." (The Brecher's nomination for the 1989 Miraculous Recovery of the Year Award).

A patient suffering from a wide range of disorders, including serious hypertension, diabetes, a variety of circulatory disorders and multiple sclerosis, and a debilitating weakness of the muscles on her right side, slurred speech, paralyzed, unable to speak, said, "It is a miracle. I feel like I did 15 years ago."

Is your doctor a "miracle worker"? "Miracles? I do not think I have any." Pose the same question to any Chelation doctor, and he'll rattle off as many detailed tales of near-death recoveries he has overseen as you have patience to hear.

More Run-Of-The-Mill Everyday 'Miracles': "If I hadn't seen this myself, I'd swear someone made it up."

"I've researched the medical literature. In every case the results of the therapy with chelating agents were just short of the fantastic."

Cause of Disease? Free Radicals!

The worst culprit of premature ageing and death is free radical activity, the pathological activity that not only disrupts every cell in the body, including nerve cells, but, as many now believe, is also the cause of all forms of life-shortening sickness. From cancer to aids, arthritis to asthma, Alzheimer's to atherosclerosis - there is evidence free radical proliferation is largely responsible for the cell and tissue damage that eventually leads to chronic degenerative disease.

Free radicals, particularly oxygen radicals, produce a cascade of free radicals, the human counterpart of the "China Syndrome" - a nuclear plant meltdown.

The most prevalent and destructive are the oxygen radicals. Anti-oxidants such as Vitamins E and C and beta carotene function as oxygen radical neutralizers.

Eventually these nasty free radicals are liable to get you - sooner rather than later - unless you beef up your internal fortification. Anti-oxidant supplementation combined with dietary changes and

---

[66]www.etext.org/Politics/Conspiracy/Cosmic.Awareness/1993.Issues/Issue_93-06

lifestyle improvements will provide you with the most reliable protection.

The Brecher's shy away from saying Chelation has a beneficial effect on almost every modern health disaster from AIDS to tension headaches, from colds to cancer.

Why?

First, here is a short list of benefits traceable to treatment: Lowered insulin requirements, lowered blood cholesterol, reduced blood pressure, normalization of cardiac arrhythmias, leg muscle cramps, allergies, weight, psychological and emotional status, sight, hearing, taste, heart contractions, varicose veins, age spots, aches and pains, arthritis, hair loss, impotence, Alzheimer's, diuretics, cold extremities, chronic fatigue, memory and concentration, post cataract vision, hair, nails, skin, wrinkles and more youthful appearance.

Second, each year this trend away from generalization to specialization grows stronger. But even if specialization were not in vogue, Chelation's cure-a-lot reputation would be a detriment. An inevitable stigma dogs any remedy that does too much, making it vulnerable to 'snake-oil' devaluation. One of the main reasons for the controversy is because it IS so successful in a variety of serious conditions. As one image-conscious doctor with a prestigious background confessed: "It is downright embarrassing to find myself endorsing a cure-all like a patent medicine side-show hawker."

Bottom line, the more Chelation cures the worse press it gets. Chelation doctors never say 'never'.

An 80 year-old lawyer Chelated for senility: "It is exhilarating to have a mate who's been sexually 'dead' for decades suddenly exhibiting sexual desires."

The younger and healthier population is adding new and exciting awareness of Chelation's potential, as these essentially well young adults report that after Chelation they think more clearly, are less sluggish, concentrate better, have fewer headaches, more energy.

"Chelation is proving to be a real solution to the 'yuppie' disease of the 1990's: chronic fatigue syndrome."

"Chelation is a potent answer to 'executive burnout'".

"Call it what you will," Dr. Ettl states, "emotional wipe-out, workaholic fatigue, professional disenchantment, the stress of success, or some similar career-related complaint, in many instances these subtle psychological symptoms are not the result of psychological dysfunction, but the adverse physical effects of a toxic environment."[67]

---

[67] As quoted in *Forty-Something Forever* by Harold and Arlene Brecher

Cancer

Projections are for one in three Westerners to suffer from one or other form of cancer. What if the incidence could be cut back to 10%, or better still, prevented? Banner headlines, prime-time documentation and a Nobel Prize? The fact is, such a discovery *has* been made. Published research suggests Chelation may well be the simple, easily available and effective countermeasure.

"But every physician who Chelates people must notice that our patients just do not get cancer."

We are not going to discuss cancer in detail in this manual, but if Cancer is a concern for you, we highly recommend *The Omega Cancer Clinic* in Tijuana Mexico, Rome Italy, and Tokyo Japan. [68]

What is a Balanced Diet?

The unmistakable truth is that the balanced diet is a myth - for all practical purposes it is nonexistent. Today's edibles grow on mineral depleted soil, are manufactured with consideration to appearance, picked before they've extracted all the nutrients necessary for their ripening and processed to last on store shelves. They have lost nutritional value every step of the way.

It is close to impossible to secure your daily nutrient and vitamin requirements from foods.

Ultimate health and longevity can only be achieved by beefing up with vitamins and minerals, and one would expect to find a wide choice of suitable products.

But beware. Our research has found that many vitamin pills are worthless. Many vitamin products either contain far less nutrition than labeled, are old and have lost potency, or have been so badly mishandled throughout the production/distribution process, a jar of jelly beans would provide more nutritional value.

A reliable source of vitamins and other effective health products is *Real Health Products.*[69]

Do not Neglect the Minerals

Recent literature review places two minerals in the spotlight: Magnesium and Potassium.

An equally prestigious cardiologist, Dr. Norman Kaplan, believes adults should consume at least 2,000 milligrams of potassium a day.[70]

The Brecher's believe there would be a significant reduction in cardiovascular disease and cancer incidence if potassium/sodium ratios

---

[68] www.omegacancerclinic.com/
[69] www.realhealthproducts.net/
[70] *Kaplan's Clinical Hypertension* by Norman M Kaplan MD

could be brought back into balance. Given the possibility of substantial and widespread potassium deficiency, it is no wonder the world is de-energizing. A potassium-deficient diet for just one week results in muscular weakness, lethargy and extreme fatigue. Muscles get flabby, intestinal mobility is reduced leading to constipation. Poor eyesight, throbbing migraine headaches, insomnia and bruises, cuts and injuries that resist healing are but a few of the more disheartening symptoms. Kidney failure and tinnitus (ringing in the ears) are also common. It can be more serious, including cardiac abnormalities and sudden death from heart attacks.

Oral Chelation

Dr. Kurt Donsbach, the Dean of Nutritional Medicine, is convinced that any compound combining all those ingredients known to reduce Free Radical activity as well as combining the specific nutrients necessary to keep heart and circulatory systems healthy, would fit the bill. You can protect yourself against the possibility of heart disease (or restore your body to normalcy if you already have such a disease) by consuming all of the nutrients the body uses to abort or neutralize explosive Free Radical action on a daily basis.

An Oral Chelate - NONI

In their book, the Brecher's recommend an oral Chelate and then go on to say that it is possible a superior concoction will emerge someday.

Well, several months ago one of the chelating physicians we have relied upon over the years called our attention to a potassium-rich liquid, NONI. He recommended it as a reliable natural means of satisfying mineral requirements and "upping" energy levels.

We take NONI for the simplest reason - we have not found anything better. We have not found anything nearly as good.

A closer study of the ingredients that make up this unique botanical formula suggests it provides much, much more. Check any recently published herbal guide and you will discover the herbs are rich in antioxidants and magnesium, all of which add up to NONI being the closest simulation yet to the oral Chelate so many have been seeking for so long a time.

The intravenous method of Chelation is preferable when heart health has deteriorated to the point where surgical intervention has been suggested, or there is some indication that free-radical pathology has progressed to a point requiring strenuous remedies.

But if your health is not that far gone, or you are seeking all-round supplementation to rejuvenate and revitalize yourself, NONI is probably the most 'user-friendly' nutritional product to be found. Its ingredients, being natural, work in harmony with each other and within the body. When herbal preparations are free of binders and fillers, more of their beneficial properties get into the bloodstream.

Studies have shown that supplements bound in a food matrix, the way nature intended, are superior to those composed of bare vitamins and minerals such as found in pharmaceutical products. Nature operates holistically - taking supplements is in some sense unnatural, but the closer they resemble a natural product, the better the prospect they will work synergistically with the body's systems to boost health. It should come as no surprise that roots, seeds and leaves have the power to heal.

So, if you are serious about your health and longevity, our ongoing research suggests that there is currently no better oral Chelate available than NONI.[71]

Chelation Summary

- Most disease is caused by Free Radicals;
- Chelation removes Free Radicals (Intravenous for life-threatening symptoms; oral for non-urgent);
- Due to the polluted environment, every Westerner needs detoxifying by Chelation;
- To maintain health, the correct nutrients and vitamins are needed;
- It is virtually impossible to obtain adequate nutrients from store-bought food;
- Pharmaceutical nutrients are often unobtainable, and are frequently not taken up by the body;
- Nutrients must be in a Food Matrix to be assimilated by the body;
- Even with an adequate supply of nutrients, the body cannot absorb them, unless it is first detoxified by Chelation;
- With proper protection from Free Radicals in the form of ongoing oral Chelation and proper foods with extra nutrients in a food matrix, an extended, active, healthy and useful life to age 120 becomes a realistic goal.
- The most effective oral Chelation supplement available today is NONI.[71]

Colon Cleansing

We now move on to the somewhat unpleasant, yet extremely necessary discussion of the removal of "mucoid or colon plaque". Without this procedure, you are severely limiting the body's absorption of the nutrients mentioned previously. This colon plaque exists in everyone,

---

[71] www.freedomtechnology.org/noni

and the extent to which it limits absorption depends on the extent of toxicity in your body.

No matter how healthy your lifestyle and eating habits, it is nigh on impossible to avoid the ingestion of toxins. You are no doubt aware of the chemicals present in most foods, the high level of heavy metals in bottled and tap water and the preservatives in all processed foods. There is evidence to suggest that the air we breathe has high concentrations of aluminum particles, chemically sprayed by aircraft over densely populated towns.[72]

These toxins, unless eliminated, line the bowels and prevent absorption of nutrients. An annual exercise is required to remove these deposits, to ensure the full benefit of NONI.

Dr. Bernard Jensen is one of the pioneers of using colon cleansing to improve a person's quality of life. In his book, *Tissue Cleansing Through Bowel Management*, Jensen describes what happens after years of toxicity build-up.

"The heavy mucus coating in the colon thickens and becomes a host of putrefaction. The blood capillaries to the colon begin to pick up the toxins, poisons and noxious debris as it seeps through the bowel wall. All tissues and organs of the body are now taking on toxic substances.

Here is the beginning of true autointoxication on a physiological level. One autopsy revealed a colon to be 9 inches in diameter with a passage through it no larger than a pencil. The rest was caked up layer upon layer of encrusted fecal material. This accumulation can have the consistency of truck tire rubber. It is that hard and black. Another autopsy revealed a stagnant colon to weigh in at an incredible 40 pounds."[73]

To put it bluntly, the "sewer system" must work properly otherwise the body remains soaking in its own putrid waste, encouraging disease processes and eluding vitality-producing and health-building forces.

But not many medical doctors are aware of this procedure, or even the benefits of the procedure.

Dr. Richard Anderson explains why in his book *Cleanse & Purify Thyself*:

"Surgeons and regular doctors are not trained in the subject of mucoid plaque and therefore remain unaware of this important bowel condition. The mucoid plaque is usually less than one-fourth of an inch in many areas of the bowel (except in heavy meat and dairy eaters). It usually develops from a semi-transparent liquid solution (mucin) and may look like it is part of the intestinal wall itself as it takes on the

[72] www.nexusmagazine.com/articles/chemtrails.html
[73] *Tissue Cleansing Through Bowel Management* by Dr. Bernard Jensen, 1981

exact shapes, striations, and bulges of the intestinal wall. Until the mucoid plaque begins to mix with fecal matter, its colon and texture may appear similar to healthy bowel mucosa. Unless one knows what they are looking for, it may be difficult to identify, especially by sight. Therefore, to doctors using endoscopy and to surgeons, it is unnoticeable unless they are familiar with the many different appearances mucoid plaque may have."[74]

How is Colon Plaque Removed?

This is a simple procedure, which should ideally be performed annually and can be done at home without the need for medical supervision. It usually consists of a week-long fast, together with the ingestion of specially formulated herbs, fiber, Bentonite clay and laxatives. The process cleanses intestinal accumulation from the entire digestive system including the stomach, small intestine and large intestine (colon).

Bentonite clay is a powder that is typically drunk five times per day after being mixed with Organic Apple juice. This formula is traditionally used for its strong absorptive properties which work powerfully to draw hardened mucus build-up and fecal matter out of the intestinal tract.

You will be required to fast during these seven days or the Bentonite clay will simply bind to the food you are eating and not the waste you are trying to remove.

The process can be additionally enhanced by introducing a Colonic Irrigation at the same time as the fast. This is a medically supervised process by which water-flow controlled by nothing more than the force of gravity is cycled through the colon to flush out the mucus build-up.

The Colon Cleansing Kit

We highly recommend Martha Volchok's *Colon Cleansing Kit for Radiant Health*. She ships internationally from the US and we have been very happy with her service and product.[75]

Colonic Irrigation

You will have to contact your own GP for a recommendation for this procedure. It can be done at home, but we highly recommend you go to a trained specialist for your first few visits.

---

[74] *Cleanse & Purify Thyself* by Dr. Richard Anderson, Christobe, 2000. See also www.cleanse.net
[75] www.marthavolchok.com/

Wrapping Up

The combined therapies of Oral Chelation and Colon Cleansing are powerful and necessary treatments in the search for Ultimate Health & Longevity.

However, as we have stated before, you will not easily find practitioners in these potent alternative health extension treatments. Expect to encounter resistance from your GP, depending on how open they are to alternative treatments. Expect to encounter many negative reports about the treatments, but bear in mind that these stories are usually linked in some way to the Medical Establishment, who stand to lose greatly if the masses were to wake up to the low-cost, effective methods available.

We recommend being fully informed before you approach your doctor. Read all of the health related resources in Appendix D on page 238 and spend some time researching online, including all the negative reports.

We want to emphasize the importance of you taking responsibility for your own health and longevity. Embracing the responsibility for your own life is the core principle of *Fresh Wisdom* and holistic living. We urge you not to hand over that responsibility to us or anyone else. Only you know what is right for you, and we trust you will take this matter of your life seriously.

~~~

And in the end, it's not the years in your life that count. It's the life in your years. – Abraham Lincoln

The young do not know enough to be prudent, and therefore they attempt the impossible -- and achieve it, generation after generation. – Pearl S. Buck

To hold the same views at forty as we held at twenty is to have been stupefied for a score of years, and take rank, not as a prophet, but as an unteachable brat, well birched and none the wiser. – Robert Louis Stevenson

Age puzzles me. I thought it was a quiet time. My seventies were interesting and fairly serene, but my eighties are passionate. I grow more intense as I age. – Florida Scott Maxwell

I'm not interested in age. People who tell me their age are silly. You're as old as you feel. – Elizabeth Arden

15. Business in the Future

In the previous Wealth Creation chapter, we discussed the concept of money and leverage. We then explained how powerful the Internet is as a tool for achieving massive leverage. We also explained that many failed with their Internet business for one of two reasons:
- Because they do not have the right product or
- Because they cannot connect with buyers for their product.

It is as simple as that.

In this chapter we are going to show you exactly how to identify hot product markets, and then how to easily create products. In the next Wealth Creation chapter we will show you how to find buyers for your product, and you will be blown away how easy it is.

You see, we have applied the concept of leverage to everything we do at Freedom Technology, including marketing on the Internet. So instead of starting with a brand new product from scratch, we plug the product into an existing proven marketing vehicle filled with thousands of thinking individuals hungry for guidance and information.

Before we discuss marketing a product on the Internet, we need to talk about business values and what you wish to achieve in your business. You will not hear any Internet Marketer who wants to sell a 'How To' Manual explain this, so take note. By understanding this section, you will quickly be able to identify the cons online, and there are *many*.

Definitions

The following definitions are adapted from *The History of Neo-Tech.*[76]

Mysticism

Mysticism is defined as:
- Any mental or physical attempt to recreate, evade, or alter reality through dishonesty, rationalizations, non sequiturs, emotions, deceptions, or force;
- Any attempt to use the mind to create reality rather than to identify and integrate reality.

Mysticism is a disease -- an epistemological disease that progressively undermines one's capacity to think, to identify reality, to live competently. Mysticism is also a collective disease that affects everyone who looks toward others, or the group, or the leader for solutions to his or her own problems and responsibilities.

The symptoms of mysticism are dishonest communication, out-of-context assertions or attacks, use of non sequiturs, rationalizations, jumbled or nonintegrated thinking -- all leading to mind-created

---

[76] www.neo-tech.com/orientation/

"realities". Those symptoms are most commonly exhibited by politicians, clergymen, union leaders, lawyers, media commentators, university professors and entertainment personalities who wish to con some value from you, instead of producing real value. Real value is produced by aggressively competitive entrepreneurs, innovators, business people and industrialists who, interestingly are often depicted as the malefactors of society by the mystics previously mentioned.

The mystic's life is basically irrational and unhappy with perhaps some scattered islands of rationality and happiness. By contrast, the non-mystic's life is basically rational and happy with perhaps some scattered islands of irrationality and unhappiness.

Turning to one's inner self, mystics find unhappiness, anxiety, and hatred. On the other hand, non-mystics find happiness, equanimity, and love.

Business

Business is defined as:

- The competitive development, production, and marketing of values that benefits others.

Any and every aspect of business succeeds to the extent that effort, thinking, planning, and action are free of mysticism...or fails to the extent that mysticism is injected into any decision. Business ultimately flourishes in the absence of mysticism or dies in the presence of mysticism. Mysticism is the creating of problems where none exist; business is the solving of problems wherever they do exist. Mysticism represents stagnation and death; business represents growth and life. Mysticism is non-business; business is non-mysticism.

Since the early days of Phoenician commerce, envious and destructive mystics have striven to besmirch the value producers, their business enterprises, and their competitive products. Legions of pseudo-intellectuals, say-much/do-little underachievers, envious non-producers, and mystic-manipulating con men, especially in the media and academe, constantly attack businesses and their creators. With unfounded accusations, the attackers imply that business people lack care, humanity, compassion or social concerns. Such implications contradict the facts. Indeed, only through business and its creators do societies advance and individuals prosper.

Laziness

The choice between exerting effort or defaulting to laziness determines the course of every human's life and ultimately entire generations and civilizations. The three choices constantly confronting every human being are to:

- exert integrated effort,

- default to camouflaged laziness, or
- act somewhere in between (the typical salaried position).

The choice to exert integrated effort or to default to camouflaged laziness is the key choice that determines the character, competence, and future of every human being. That crucial choice must be made by everyone, continually, throughout life. ...That key choice determines the:

- Direction of an infant's life beginning at the first moment of consciousness;
- Development of a child's implicit nascent philosophy which determines that child's developing psychology;
- Development of an adult's implicit and explicit philosophy which develops that person's psychology to determine the quality of his or her life;
- Philosophies that guide entire nations, eras, and civilizations with the resulting cultures, economies, and degrees of enlightenment or darkness;
- Evolvement or regression of human consciousness, power, prosperity, happiness, and love;
- Prosperous survival or eventual destruction of human life on this planet.

Those choosing to live through automatic laziness survive by usurping or attacking values produced by others. Those usurpers and attackers include essentially all politicians and theologians as well as many dishonest professionals, attorneys, psychologists, academics, elitists, journalists, philosophers.

Well-known usurpers and attackers of values include Plato, Hitler, Stalin, FDR, the Pope, Al Capone, Pol Pot, Fidel Castro, Ralph Nader, and Jesse Helms. In addition, research shows that Einstein was a plagiarist, (particularly of his famous equation $E=mc^2$), and cheat of the highest order. While working at the U.S. government patent office he would read all the great inventions of the day before they were published. Many of them were claimed as his own.[77] Thomas Edison is also incorrectly credited with many inventions originated by Nikola Tesla.[78]

By contrast, those who choose to live through integrated effort can thrive by producing or building values for others. Those producers include working people, business people, industrialists, scientists as well as honest professionals, artists, musicians, philosophers.

---

[77] www.nexusmagazine.com/articles/einstein.html
[78] file:///lucidwork/lucidcafe/library/96feb/edison.html

Well-known value producers include Aristotle, Ray Kroc, Henry Ford, Pierre S. du Pont, Andrew Carnegie, Jay Gould, Galileo, Michelangelo, Beethoven, Nikola Tesla and Ayn Rand.

The choice between laziness and effort determines if one becomes an unhappy destroyer of values or a happy producer of values.

The Freedom Technology Business Philosophy

The reason we are explaining our business philosophy is because we are hoping that you will become interested in using our services to market something of value which you will create. We will discuss this in more detail shortly.

As you can probably guess from the previous definitions, the Freedom Technology Business Philosophy is one of:

- Using the mind to create, explain, expound on or simplify reality;
- Create value from which others can benefit;
- Embrace the exertion of disciplined, integrated effort to produce real value.

This philosophy flies in the face of almost every Internet Marketer, who will convince you to find other people's content to build your site (laziness), or build sites which attract traffic and then provide Google Adsense Ads (no value creation). No wonder the Internet is in the state it is currently.

By producing real value in the form of original digital downloadable products (eBooks, videos, training manuals, etc) you are immediately differentiating yourself and setting yourself up for long-term success.

The intention is to use existing successful products and overlay the effective Freedom Technology principles to create something useful and of real value. You create the product and we market it for you. You can even do this while enjoying the security of a guaranteed income (while you are still employed). As the results from your efforts exceed your salary, you can confidently leave your job to create even more products, and thus increase your revenue.

As an example, consider the hugely successful *Chicken Soup for the Soul* marketing vehicle. While millions of copies have been sold (already over 75 million!), the concepts explained therein are, shall we say, rather bland. Imagine following the same marketing recipe for success, while expounding the Freedom Technology principles – the result could be phenomenal. Not only in terms of income generated, but the effect on an entire generation or more.

Finding the Right Product

The absolute key to your success anytime you decide to begin any money-making project online is effective market research. Market Research is where all big profits begin. In contrast, without market research, your failure online is almost guaranteed.

Everyone has their own methods for conducting market research, but we are going to reveal to you five key questions to ask about every market before taking action on a project. We are also going to show 4 free highly effective market research tools. The following section is taken from The Reese Report.[79]

Five Keys to Effective Market Research

Notice that the word "effective" is included as part of this section's title.

Anyone can do research online, but unless you know how to properly tie all of that research together into usable information that reveals whether or not you should proceed with a project idea, you are simply wasting your time. Here are the five keys to effective market research:

1. **Is The Market Already Buying Something Similar?** Many people teach Internet Marketing beginners to start off by promoting something they have an interest in... a hobby, profession, talent, etc. This is not an effective business strategy because regardless of how much you enjoy something, it is pointless to build a web site and try to earn a living from something if people are not buying what you are selling. Now, there is nothing wrong with building a site on something just as a hobby, but if you are wanting to build a business, the first key is to figure out what people are spending their money on, and then build a business around a related product or service. It matters little that you absolutely *hate* a certain type of product. If you find that people are interested in that product, and more importantly, willing to spend their hard earned money for that product, you need to find a way to get in on the action. Remember, it is not what you like that matters. It is what your potential customers like that matters.

2. **Is The Market Big Enough?** Using tools to do keyword research is an effective way of establishing the number of searches done any given month for a certain keyword phrase. These tools include the *Overture Search Term Suggestion Tool* (Yahoo now calls it their Keyword Selector Tool)[80]and

---

[79] *The Reese Report* by John Reese, www.reesereport.com
[80] http://inventory.overture.com/

Wordtracker.[81] The ideal is to target keywords which enjoy between 10,000 and 20,000 searches per month. The point is that you want the market to be large enough that you are able to have enough exposure for you to determine whether or not your idea is worth all of the effort.

3. **Can I Reach The Market Cost-Effectively?** Apart from waiting for and relying on unreliable free search engine traffic, the most common form of marketing online is Pay-Per-Click, in which you bid for the placement of adverts on websites. Every click on your ad generates a targeted visitor and will cost you anything from a few cents up to hundreds of dollars. It does not do you any good to go into a market where you have to buy clicks for $20-40/click unless you are selling a product for thousands of dollars. You have to keep your click costs below 30 or 40 cents for a $30 or $40 eBook, for example. Otherwise, you simply are not going to make a profit no matter how good your conversions are, for the most part.

4. **Are There Multiple "Back Door" Markets That Connect To The Market?** This next step is the exception to the rules that your market has to be big enough, and that your marketing must be cost-effective. The idea of "back door" markets consists of directing people to products or other resources that, on the surface, appear totally unrelated to the original product or market, but are also consumed by or purchased by a prospect that is active in that certain niche. For example, how similar are golf and travel insurance? They are not similar, are they? Well, the idea is to think about what other markets "connect" to your target market, create sub-sites for those other markets, and then link to them from your original site. Then, as you think of other back door markets related to those sub-sites, you can make sites for those markets, and before you know it, you have a chain of sites that seem unrelated on the surface, but allow your prospects to lead themselves along that chain, gratifying their needs and wants along the way.

Let us say you create a site about golf. Obviously, other sites related to golf like golf courses, golf clubs, and so on would make sense, but what about golf vacations? Did you know that people actually take vacations strictly to play golf? That being the case, does not it also make sense that these people who are wanting to go on golf vacations may also need some travel insurance for their trips? If you were to create separate sites for each of those keywords, just think of all the possibilities for other sites that could branch off from this little

---

[81] www.wordtracker.com/

network. By using "back door" markets, you may turn a site that initially does not make much, if any, profit because the market is not big enough, or because you paid too much for advertising, into a profitable entry way into a successful network of web sites. Brainstorm a little and see if there are some back door markets that you might be able to tie into the markets you are currently promoting to.

5. **Are There Existing Partners In The Market?** Competition on the Internet is not only a good thing, it is a great thing. If you create your own products, you want partners who you can sell your products through. By setting up an affiliate program and finding related businesses who would like to offer your products to their customers and/or prospects, you are leveraging the traffic that these partners are generating.

Market Research Tools

eBay

One of the most effective free places to conduct market research when you begin a new project is at eBay[82]. When considering selling some sort of product, you can usually find that product or topic on eBay.

If you visit eBay you will notice the "Categories" section on the left side of the page. This is an excellent place to start if you are looking for related sites to add to your back door markets for some of your products.

By using eBay, and other big companies on the Internet, you are exercising the principle of leverage, because they have already done all of the research for you.

They have huge teams of people who are trained to research different markets and drill down as deep as possible to find all the related segments of those markets.

For instance, if you click on "antiques" under the categories section on eBay, you will see a whole list of subcategories, each with its own list of even more precise categories.

One way of looking at it is that "antiques", for example, is the generic keyword, and each subcategory, such as "Asian antiques", are more precise keywords or specific niches.

How to Find the Hottest Items in Any Market

eBay can also tell you which items are most in demand by their web site visitors. By tapping into this valuable information, you can create information products geared towards these hungry markets.

---

[82] www.ebay.com

Let us go back to the "antiques" example from above. Once you click on the antiques link under "categories", find the section on the web page entitled, "Category Community Links". Then click the link that says "Read the latest Seller Newsletter".

Next, notice the "New and Improved Hot List" section. Click on the "Hot List" link within that paragraph. You can go into this area and you will discover trends and analysis for different types of products within each of the main subcategories, including the hot search terms.

This information is fantastic for determining the hottest topics to create information products for.

Yahoo

Yahoo is another example of a huge company that has spent thousands of man hours on researching the thousands of markets available to us, and we are going to show you how to profit from the work they have already done for you.

If you visit their web site[83], you will see the different categories listed on their home page.

By clicking on the "Real Estate" category, you will be able to tell within seconds exactly what people are looking for when it comes to real estate.

Notice all of the links within the column that appears on the left side of the page. These links are exactly what people are looking for... how to sell a home, rent an apartment, loans, refinancing, homeowner's insurance, and on and on.

Let us look at another category... "Health".

If you scroll down the page that comes up, there is a section that offers different Yahoo Groups that you can join in order to get in touch with others who are concerned with certain topics.

The six categories they have listed, currently alternative medicine, depression, diabetes, fitness & nutrition, pregnancy, and weight issues, are the health related issues that are the most searched for or discussed within Yahoo's interactive groups.

If you decide that you want to create an information product on health related issues, these six topics are definitely subjects you will want to cover.

Everything that you find on this health page, or any page for any other category, gives you clues as to exactly what topics are hot right now with consumers.

Currently, there is a poll on the health page that asks for people's main skin issue concerns, and out of about 5600 total votes, acne is the biggest concern (33%).

---

[83] www.yahoo.com

You can find this information by clicking on "View Results Without Voting" which appears within the poll box.

With maybe 10 seconds of research from the time it took to visit Yahoo, click on "health", and click on the "View Results…" link, you now have some key information that will help determine what type of information product you should consider. Obviously we are just using these categories as examples of how the system works.

Go back to Yahoo's main page and click on "Financing". Do you think that all of the categories and subcategories that appear along the left column of that page might be what people are most interested in when it comes to investing and personal finance?

We cannot emphasize enough how powerful this web site can be for you and your business. Yahoo, eBay, and even Google are amazing tools that allow you to develop profitable online businesses, and to think that they have been right under our noses the entire time.

Google Zeitgeist

This is a fantastic little tool that "exposes interesting trends, patterns, and surprises", according to their web site[84].

This site shows what searches have increased in frequency the most during a given week, as well as those searches that have declined the most in a given week.

Another great feature with this tool is that you can see what the most popular search terms are for various categories, such as popular women, popular men, popular brick & mortar companies, popular travel queries, etc.

You can also see what the most popular sports, video games, and cars are, for example, in terms of which items are searched for the most.

You definitely want to keep your eye on this site to keep your thumb on the pulse of what people are searching for on a weekly basis.

Another cool feature of this site is their archived section of trends over the last few years. You can click on "2001", for example, to see what people were searching for, and you will be able to correlate those searches with the trends that were hot at the time.

Although this is a great little tool for pinpointing different trends, you want to be careful not to create full blown businesses based on trends alone because trends usually become money makers and not long-term businesses.

---

[84] www.google.com/press/zeitgeist.html

GoogSpy

You can use this fantastic tool to spy on your competitors in order to find out what keywords they are bidding on at Google Adwords.

But you can also use GoogSpy[85] to have your competitors show you what other markets you should be considering.

Simply type in a term into the search box, click on one of the keywords that the results give you and it will give you the URLs of the sites that are buying Adwords for those keywords.

You can then click on one of these URLs to discover all of the keywords that that company is bidding on.

In this way you can "borrow" keyword ideas from your competitors, but for our purposes, we want to look at all of these other keywords these companies are using, and think about all the different markets these keywords represent.

For example, let us use the example of "corvette", click on "corvette engines", click on the first URL that comes up, and we find that this company is bidding on dozens of keywords.

Some of these keywords include jeep engine, mini cooper parts, superchargers, and so on.

If you are thinking about creating an information product related to corvettes, you could come up with some other ideas for related sites.

Also, there is a list of that company's biggest competitors along the left column of the page. You can click on each one of these company's URLs and repeat the process to develop even more ideas for information products.

So not only can you develop a large number of keywords to use in your marketing as a result of using this tool, you can also develop a whole list of other markets that you can create information products for.

Wordtracker

You no longer have to guess which markets are the most lucrative online. While this is not a free tool, Wordtracker[86] is by far the best research tool to discover niche markets which you can advertise to. Use this tool to establish exactly how many people searched for a particular keyword phrase in the last 2 months. It even suggests related searches. We will not provide examples of how to use this tool here, because they have a detailed User Guide. If you are really serious about your research, this is one tool worth having – try it for a day or week to get an idea of the power behind this excellent tool.

---

[85] www.googspy.com/
[86] www.wordtracker.com

How to Create Your Product & Run Your Business

The real secret to building wealth online is creating a powerful 'organization'. A perfect example of this is Michael Green's *How To Corporation*[87]. If you visit that site you will see a huge range of products, all supposedly generated by one person. But "Michael Green" is in fact a pen-name for a hugely successful British publishing empire which generates significant revenue for their small family-run business.

But do not panic. We are not suggesting that the key to making the big money online is to go and lease an expensive office and put 60 people on a payroll.

However, until you can learn to leverage the time and resources of others, you will never make as much as you possibly can, or reach as many people as you possibly can. That is just a fact, and is one of the core principles of Freedom Technology.

There is one proven fact that will never go away no matter what – you only have so many hours in a day that you can work on your business. Even if you do not go to sleep that is still 24 hours. You will never be able to work 25 hours in a single day – trust us, we have tried.

Because of this time limitation, how do you make more money in your business (regardless of what stage it is currently at) if your time is limited?

It is easy. You must leverage the time of others. You must embrace (and effectively utilize) the ability to outsource. In order for you to make maximum cash from your efforts, you absolutely – positively - must start outsourcing. You must build and run your profit-making organization by leveraging other people.

Outsourcing

The best way to start building your organization is to start by using just one other person to do something for your business. You can hire this person to do some work as a freelancer, and only pay them when you need work done.

A great example of this is to hire someone anytime you need web pages designed and created. Maybe you are already creating web pages yourself. If so, we strongly recommend you stop doing it.

Why? There is no money in it.

Pay someone $100 to make a site for you and use the time you saved from doing it yourself to work on your product creation or marketing. Remember, marketing is where the real money is made – not creating web sites, doing programming, creating cute graphics, etc.

---

[87] www.howtocorp.com

You can go to elance.com[88] or rentacoder.com[89] and find plenty of freelancers who will do a wide variety of things for you. You can also do a Google[90] search for "freelance XXXX" (substituting XXXX with designer, programmer, writer, etc.) and you can find many people that way.

So, if all you do is find someone you can pay every now and then when you need web design work done, you have freed up many hours of your time for you to put into your business. This is a great place to start.

The small amount you will pay for someone to do that grunt work for you will more than pay for itself.

The second thing you should be looking to outsource is HTML programming. Do not even think about learning any of this nerd code. Or, you might already be a programmer yourself. But, guess what? There is no money in it. Again, it is all about the marketing. Find a freelance programmer who can do some work for you when you need it - such as working with your shopping cart, creating a custom autoresponder script, or anything else you need programming for.

You should be noticing a trend with what we are saying. Pay someone only when you need the work done. That means do not go hiring someone full-time. In most cases that is just idiotic.

If you hired a construction team to build a house for you, are you going to keep paying them after the house is built? Of course not. Internet marketing is the same way. It is made up of web pages, some programming (if necessary), and content. That is basically it.

All of those things are created one time and produce results for a long time. There is no reason to keep paying someone after something has been created. You only pay them if you want something NEW created.

Ghost Writing

The next type of person (or people) you need to hire to do work for you are ghostwriters. These are people who will write content on your behalf, but still allow you to market the product as your own.

The Internet is based on content. You have to have it for your web pages, your autoresponder series, your newsletter issues, your articles, etc. Much of this you can pay a talented writer to research and write for you – for practically any market imaginable.

Writing is not only very time consuming, but for many people it is a dreaded task. So, why not just pay someone to create content for you that you will use for your marketing or your info product?

---

[88] www.elance.com
[89] www.rentacoder.com
[90] www.google.com

Once again, if you do this, you will be freeing up more of your time. This gives you more time that you could be spending on marketing your business or creating additional product ideas.

Customer Support

The next thing you should strongly consider outsourcing - and for many this will be the first thing - is customer support.

If you have a business that requires customer support (i.e., your customers email and call with problems, or need refunds, or just want to complain, etc.), you need to run, not walk, to outsource your customer support.

Almost every business has customer support tasks (if not all of them) that can be outsourced. You can train someone one time to handle certain problems, and they will always be able to handle them for you.

Ninety-nine percent of your customer support requests will be duplicate requests you will receive from customer to customer. Unless you absolutely love to handle your own customer support (which if true you are probably insane!), you should look to outsource it. We highly recommend workaholics4hire.com[91]. They are currently handling the customer support for many online marketers – and doing a fantastic job. They will take really good care of you and your business.

Another huge benefit of outsourcing your customer support is that you will not be faced with any negativity that comes from complaining customers, refund requests, etc.

You obviously want to keep up with the feedback of your customers so you can address certain things that need to be changed or improved. But, many complaints will be the same - and you reading more than one copy of those complaints is not going to do you any good. In fact, it can harm your productivity.

For example, every business that sells a product or service is going to experience refunds. That is just the nature of the business. No matter how great your product is there will always be a small percentage of people who want their money back.

There is no question about it, you will take it personally each time someone requests a refund. It reminds you that someone was not happy with your product – even though studies have shown that 90% of refund requests come from people who made up their minds to return a product even before they purchased it.

So, if you outsource your customer support, you will not be seeing all these refund requests. The service handling your support will just promptly issue the refund and take care of that customer. Trust us when we say that by not being faced with every single refund request,

---

[91] www.workaholics4hire.com/

you will make more money. By not being faced with that negativity, it will make you much happier and allow you to focus on more positive aspects of your business.

That reason alone is why you should outsource your customer support ASAP if you are trying to handle it yourself.

There are many other things you should be outsourcing in your business – accounting, legal, tax preparation, product fulfillment, and more. And the main reason for you to outsource as much as you possibly can is simple. It is so you can focus all of your time and effort on what you want to do. If you structure your organization properly, you can focus on those tasks and leave the rest of the "operations" to others.

It does not matter if you are just starting out with a brand new, tiny business with a tiny budget, or you are trying to grow a business that is already making millions. The principles are the same and you need to understand them. The reason why we want to make sure you fully understand the concept of building your organization is because that will truly allow you to build wealth with your business.

Most people marketing online are doing everything themselves. This is a huge mistake. For pennies on the dollar, you can have other people helping you do things for your business that will allow you to put more time into the things that bring in the big profits.[92]

Connecting with Buyers

Now that you have created a killer information product which adds real value to others, the next challenge is to connect your product with people hungry for that information. We will not kid you – this is not an easy task. There is an entire science behind generating targeted traffic to your website, and to make matters worse, the algorithms are constantly changing. Staying on top of the latest trends is a full time endeavor.

But that is where Freedom Technology comes in. In the next and final Wealth Creation chapter we will explain exactly how our unique and rather effective concept will assist you in connecting your product with people hungry for your information. This is another way in which you can outsource a critical part of your business.

If you *are* interested in finding out about the science behind getting traffic to your website, we can highly recommend Michael Green's *How to Promote a Product Online*.[93]

We hope you are staring to get a sense of how powerful the Internet can be. It is a passion for us, and we hope will become one for you too.

---

[92] Extracted and adapted from *The Reese Report* by John Reese, www.reesereport.com
[93] www.howtocorp.com/sales.php?offer=mbh66&pid=22

16. The Biblical World View and Man's Purpose

In Chapter 10 - How Religion Affects Our World View on page 70, we discussed the con of man made religions, and the Laws of Metaphysical Truths, which are:

- The Universe and the mind of man were brought into existence out of nothing - or out of something which is currently beyond the ability of our mind to comprehend - by an Initiator outside of this world system.
- At the Universal Level, there are Two Opposing Forces in existence, and these can be broadly defined as Positive and Negative. The positive force is naturally good (love), and the negative force is naturally evil (death).
- The Negative Force is temporary – with only the Positive Force eventually remaining, resulting in a dimension of Metaphysical Love.

In Chapter 12 - The Fresh Wisdom Ethos on page 101, we built on those principles and explained the Freedom Technology Ethos and Mission. We also explained that we apply a Biblical World View, which is the only scientifically (empirically) proven, sustainable and viable World View that has no inconsistencies. We summarized the Biblical World View as follows:

- **The Universe** was created by an Outside-Of-This-System Initiator at a specific point and identifiable time, in keeping with known laws which are currently in use to determine things like space trajectories of interplanetary craft, microwave transmissions, etc.
- **The Purpose** for which Man was also created and put into this System is for Training: Training in understanding and control of the Universe and dealing with the 2 forces of positive and negative that are inherent in the system, commonly called 'good' and 'evil'. An additional purpose is for future E5 Management Tasks - we will have specific 'jobs' in the next dimension.
- **The Solution** for this 'Good and Evil' or Positive/Negative Conflict is provided by Initiator. The resolution of the problem of the existence of 'evil' is not achieved by Man, but supplied extraneously (from outside the system) by Initiator. Recognition of this is part of the training and comes for all at some point. For some it is given to them to understand now in the E4 and for the others, it will be given later in E5. In other words: All will eventually understand fully, when (in Initiator's own time) their eyes are opened by Initiator (and no-one else, although humans can plant seeds).

- **The Future**: There IS another (provable) Dimension (E5) in which Time is not a limiting factor. All human beings DO appear into this dimension – it is an inherent (automatic) outcome of the Created Order. This present order is merely an interim state of preparation; similar to the birth of a child after being nurtured in the womb (E4) and coming into the world (E5).

We are now going to delve a little deeper into why we place so much emphasis on a Biblical World View. In short, apart from being scientifically proven, it is also the only World View which provides true purpose and meaning for our life on earth.

We are also establishing the reliability of this source document so that we can make the next 'Quantum Leap' based upon these Scriptures – that of reaching The Omega Point.

Even if you are familiar with the Bible, we challenge you to read this chapter with a totally open mind. You may find by the end of this section that your World View is currently Religious (for example Christian), instead of Biblical. There is a very important difference – read on.

What is the Bible?

Written over 1500 years, completed 2000 years ago, it has stood the test of time – the greatest test of all literature, read more than any other book by people of widely differing cultures.

Written by diverse people in different countries, from all walks of life and social positions, as history, theology, poetry, philosophy, adventure, travel and romance, it has a coherence and internal agreement that only a determined fool could deny.

The Bible's Power and Effect

During the British Coronation Ceremony a Bible is presented to the Monarch with the words:

> *"We present you with this Book, the most valuable thing this world affords. Here is wisdom. This is the Royal Law. These are the living oracles of God."*[94]

This book has the power to reform and transform, giving purpose and hope, peace and assurance of an ongoing life into another dimension. Supernatural in origin, eternal in duration, inexhaustible in meaning, personal in application and powerful in effect. It is given to us in this Dimension and will be open, or fully understood, in the next dimension (E5).

---

[94] www.byfaith.co.uk/paulbible.htm

Come to it with awe. Read it with reverence, frequently, slowly and prayerfully. And without the interference of religions.

What is the Bible About?

The Bible, with the obfuscation of religion removed, deals with every experience of life. It gives advice and help, instruction and warning, comfort and hope, correction and direction, predictions and promises.

It is a communication from the Outside-of-our-System Initiator of the Universe and recounts His materialization into this dimension (E4), with sufficient proofs to convince even the most ardent skeptic of His existence and interest in We-The-People.

In vivid terms it presents a Message, by the impact of His appearing here, of an ongoing existence into another Dimension. It is much more than a book. It is much more than a religion. It may give you hope for the future, peace of mind and an assurance of a renewed existence on into the 5th Dimension.

Or it may not. Ironically, Initiator's decision on whether to reveal understanding of the Bible to you within this dimension or not depends on His purposes for your specific life.

It is a message of a relationship, an introduction to the reality of love and another plane of existence. It may be His plan to 'tag' you now, or later. But He has given indication that He *will* do it sometime. All you can do is wait until He does make contact.

*"**You did not choose me, but I chose you** and appointed you to go and bear fruit – fruit that will last."* (emphasis added)[95]

That is very different to what many religions teach, is it not?

*"For just as the Father raises the dead and gives them life, even so the Son gives life **to whom he is pleased to give it.**"* (emphasis added)[96]

The corollary of this statement is that there are some He chooses *not* to give the understanding to.

In the meantime it makes sense to become acquainted with this work, as it is His primary way of 'tagging' people. But no matter if you are not impelled to it right now. It is just not your time…. yet.

Relax.

Evidence is that He does all things well, timeously and is absolutely in control of every aspect of the Universe, this world, its history, rulers and progress, and yours included.

Believe it or not.

It has had the most profound impact upon so many millions of people, over such an extended period of time, that to deny its Metaphysical Source is the height of irrationality. It is the ultimate

---

[95] John 15:16
[96] John 5:21

scientific evidence of a Mind greater than the whole, with purpose, even for your individual existence. You fit into a plan.

Upon reflection it may become evident to you that you are His greatest masterpiece. And a relationship with Him is on the cards, in due time.

This Book is a story of His opening up of Himself to We-The-People, both to individuals and nations, as pertinent to our modern world as it was to every age since the beginning. It is not at variance with any proven scientific fact and shows an internal concordance of knowledge of the world of science which the initial writers could not have had, except for its inspiration by an Outside Mind.[97]

It is not primarily a book of philosophy and nowhere does it argue the existence of 'God'. Yet the Initiator it reveals has been known in a personal way by many of the greatest minds that have ever lived. It speaks to every man from the simplest to the most sophisticated, at his own level of understanding.

The theme is of a gigantic Cosmic conflict between positive and negative influences. It shows the unfolding of the ultimate triumph of 'good', in the form of love. This relationship leads, via personal development, to another reality of co-existence, participation and partnership.

As the proofs of past foretelling of events and their fulfillment have been evidence of His control, so future events will be demonstrated to tie in with the predicted in such a way as to leave absolutely no doubt of the inter-connectedness within, and the reality of, the Quantum Spectrum and its evidence of pre-planning and ordering of the Universe, by an Outside-of-the-System Initiator.

You have been introduced to Him - Jesus Christ, the Passionate. Get to know him better through His unique Message to You, His Greatest Miracle.

Discover your real self.

Welcome to Ultimate Reality.

You are approaching The Omega Point.

"I came that they may have and enjoy life, and have it in abundance (to the full, till it overflows)."[98]

Let us delve into this a little deeper to see what this all means.

The Bible Code

You may be familiar with the controversy surrounding *The Bible Code*. Much of the debate is caused by Drosnin's claim that the code can be used to predict future events.

---

[97] See www.bibleandscience.com - The Institute for Biblical and Scientific Studies
[98] John 10:10 (Amplified)

The professors involved in the research for the book have made public statements supporting the existence of codes in the Bible, but denying that these codes can be used to predict the future.[99]

The controversy aside, we have included extracts from *The Bible Code* by Michael Drosnin to show the reliability of the *science* within the Bible.

"I have tried to deal with this story the way I have dealt with every other story as an investigative reporter: I've spent 5 years checking out the facts. Nothing is taken on faith.

"The Bible was encoded with information about the past and the future in a way that was mathematically beyond chance, and found in no other text.

"The scientists... the Pentagon code-breaker, the 3 referees at the math journal, the professors at Harvard, Yale and Hebrew University all started out skeptics, and ended up believers.

"There is no way within the known laws of mathematics to explain seeing the future. What we are talking about here is some intelligence that stands outside.

"In the end, all conventional science, indeed all conventional concepts of reality, may be irrelevant. If some being that stands outside the system, outside our 3 dimensions, outside of time, encoded the Bible, the code may not obey any of our laws, scientific or otherwise.

"I went to see Israel's most famous mathematician, Robert J Aumann. He is one of the world's experts in game theory and a member of both the Israeli and the US National Academy of Science.

"'The Bible code is simply fact,' said Aumann. 'It is not just Kosher, its Glatt Kosher.... There has been nothing like it in all the hundreds of years of modern science.'

"Einstein's 'theory of relativity' is also encoded. In fact, the full understanding of the Universe that eluded him, the Unified Field Theory, may also have been encoded 3,000 years ago. With his name, and again with the 'theory of relativity', the code gives the same clue: 'Add a fifth part.'

"Apparently the answer that Einstein was seeking will be found not in our 3 dimensions of space, or in his 4th dimension of time, but in the 5th dimension that all quantum physicists now agree exists." [100]

"The most ancient religious texts," noted Rips, "also state that there is a 5th dimension. They call it 'a depth of good and a depth of evil'."

---

[99] www.despatch.cth.com.au/Articles_V/Torah_Extracts.htm

[100] Extracts from *The Bible Code* by Michael Drosnin, New York: Simon & Schuster, 1997.

Prophecy, of course is not unique to the code. It happens all through the Bible.

In fact, Jack Miles in his Pulitzer Prize-winning biography of God states, "It is the miracle of prediction - fortune-telling at an international level - rather than any battlefield miracle, that is expected to bring everyone to the worship of the true God."[101]

Predictive Power Affirms Cosmic Creation

Scientists focus enormous effort on turning detections (observations and measurements) into predictions.

- Meteorologists use data to predict temperatures, wind, and precipitation;
- Astronomers use data to predict meteor showers and eclipses;
- Physicists use data to predict the existence of fundamental particles;
- Seismologists use data to predict volcanic eruptions and earthquakes.

How do they do it?

The answer gives fresh significance to a familiar and (for some) favorite childhood pastime: model building.

Predictions serve as a model's proving grounds. Major predictive failures suggest the need for major overhauls. Minor ones suggest the need for refinements. Inconsistencies indicate the presence of variables and interrelationships not yet accounted for.

One of the biggest and most challenging modeling projects yet attempted by science endeavors to depict the realities of the cosmos. A diverse array of models underwent construction and testing during the twentieth century. Major predictive failures sent most to the scrap heap.

One set of models, however, remains in the refinement process:
Hot Big Bang Models

This development comes as good news to some people, but bad news to others, because it carries implications for religious beliefs and values.

Models exist not in isolation but in relation to other models. The cosmological model demonstrates this point. It puts constraints on the models for their component parts, such as the models for star formation and life origins.

At the same time, the cosmological model either reinforces or contradicts the models into which it fits as a component part, such as the philosophical-theological models popularly known as World Views.

---

[101] *God: A Biography* by Jack Miles, Vintage, 1996

Some of the latest discoveries about the Universe, specifically about the hot big bang model, speak volumes about the predictive power of a Bible-based, science-affirming perspective on the cosmos.

This model asserts that a transcendent intelligent Creator purposefully brought the Universe into existence 'in the beginning', determined its physical laws and characteristics, and fine-tuned its development to create a home for human civilization. The hot big bang set of models closely matches these assertions.

Any breakthroughs corroborating and refining the hot big bang model, in essence, corroborate the distinctively Biblical theistic worldview.

For scientists who thrive on the corroboration and refinement phase of model building, and for anyone fascinated by this particular world view, the hot big bang model discoveries give as much cause for jubilation as a freshly painted model airplane about to be hung from a ceiling.

One such scientist who is taking model-building to the extreme is the inorganic research chemist, Dr. Frank R. Wallace[102], who plans on building a public walk-through glass model that illustrates – via interactive audio and video – an integration of vast amounts of raw physical, statistical and mathematical information currently available. The display is due for completion towards the end of this decade and will visually transform information concerning space-and-time distributions, quantities, properties and uses of the elements on quantum, macro and cosmic levels. If successful, Dr. Wallace's model will further shatter any evolution myths.

Could it be that such a model will be the Conscious Messenger for our Universe, just as Galileo's telescope was the Starry Messenger for our Solar System four centuries ago?

The Creation Model Stands Strong

Ancient contributors to Scripture, including Job, Moses, David, Solomon, Isaiah, Jeremiah, and Zechariah described various features of the big bang Universe with amazing, even supernatural, accuracy. They detailed the Universe's singular transcendent ancient beginning (from beyond matter, energy, space, and time), its ongoing expansion, the fine-tuning of its expansion, the fixity of its physical laws, and the specific and meticulous preparation for human life.

These Bible authors wrote thousands of years before Albert Einstein's equations and demonstrated cosmic expansion from a transcendent event. They wrote thousands of years before astronomers studied Type IA supernovae, measured deuterium abundances, mapped

---

[102] www.neo-tech.com/

acoustical peaks in the cosmic background radiation, measured the gravity holding together hot intergalactic gas clouds, or determined the light travel time from ancient hot and cold spots in the background radiation to the present day.

The predictive power of the Biblically based cosmic creation model attests to the divine inspiration of Scripture, thus the trustworthiness of its central message and the good news of humanity's redemption from sin through the life, death, and resurrection of Jesus Christ.

This message casts the model in the context of God's larger-than-cosmic plan for humankind.

Quantum Mechanics

Quantum Mechanics[103] is a theory in physics which primarily tries to explain the behavior of extremely small bodies, such as atoms and molecules. Scientists generally agree that it is an accurate and successful theory, and it has important applications in today's world as all electronic devices depend on Quantum Mechanics in some way. It is also important in understanding how large objects such as stars and even the entire Universe operate the way they do. The predictions of Quantum Mechanics have never been disproven after a century's worth of experiments.

The foundations of Quantum Mechanics were established during the first half of the 20th century by, among others, Max Planck, Albert Einstein, Niels Bohr, Werner Heisenberg, Erwin Schrödinger, Max Born, John von Neumann, Paul Dirac and Wolfgang Pauli.

It is the underlying framework of many fields of physics and chemistry, including condensed matter physics, quantum chemistry, and particle physics.

The cumulative evidence of Quantum Mechanics is now sufficient to rule out all theological options but one - the Bible's.

Evolution

Any discussion of World Views must deal with so-called Evolution, since this theory is blasted at us almost daily from all media sources.

The very fact that we are bombarded with this religious view by the controlled media means, to a *Fresh Thinker*, that it needs investigation.

Historical Development of Evolution

The history of Western thought brought about a rift between science and ethics. There has been an attempt to discredit creation, which was

---

[103] http://en.wikipedia.org/wiki/Quantum_mechanics

rooted in the need to deny God's existence. Thus a new 'religion' developed, postulating a 'natural' rather than an Initiator-created Universe.

Accordingly, it can be shown that any leaning towards promoting the evolutionary view requires far more faith, (since its theories are impossible to be supported by modern science) than creation requires.

Evolution is thus a competing 'god', defended quite as vehemently as any other 'religion', while unable to be proven.

Our concept of human origins thus affects the whole way we relate to the cosmos. It governs our thoughts about the future.

Creationism derives its origin from the Scriptures and is the most reasonable scientific explanation.

Evolution has arisen as an attempt to separate science from ethics, allowing ideas to be accepted which would not be possible if Creation were proven. It has thus become a desperate human (as opposed to Biblical) cause to deny God.

Thus, upon the religion of evolution, the role of science has developed into the ultimate god, in the hope that one day science will dispel all mystery, including God, the ultimate mystery.

The proper human response to mystery should be wonder instead of rebellion. Science has a major role to play in feeding religious faith, by awakening a sense of awe.

"The mystery of the kingdom of God" proclaimed by Jesus[104] has a material aspect; which an investigative, rational approach to the world, is uncovering.

Clarity of thinking in this remarkable Universe can only open the mind and heart to wonder, whereas evolution would restrain the religiously enslaved mind from knowing God better.

As the author William Harwood explains, "Insanity is a neurological dysfunction that prevents the brain from rejecting conclusions that are incompatible with the evidence."[105]

Or stated differently: only an insane person believes that evolution is a provable explanation for the existence of the Universe. The mountain of scientific evidence proves the reliability of this source document conclusively.

With the foundation thus firmly in place, it is time to make the next 'Quantum Leap' based upon these Scriptures. If nothing we have discussed thus far has fazed you, you might be in for a shock. Once again, listen carefully for the 'ring of truth'. Truth has its own distinctive sound.

And maybe this is your time to be 'tagged'.

---

[104] Mark 4:11

[105] www.neo-tech.com/pax-b1/c3.php

The Grand Affair

"Happiness can be found neither in ourselves nor in external things, but in God and in ourselves as united to Him."[106]

Romantic Love

We are going to be talking a little more about Relationships in this section, which is extracted and adapted from *The Journey of Desire* by John Eldridge.

In previous chapters on Relationships, we were consciously negative about the union between a man and a woman. This is not because we do not value relationships. On the contrary, romantic love is one of life's most important and practical achievements: Romantic love is a major source of personal growth, efficient living, happiness, joy, and pleasure. All we were trying to do is break free from previously limiting belief in preparation for *this* discussion on the Grand Affair.

Three types of love exist:
1. Sexual romantic love,
2. Nonsexual friendship and family love, and
3. Intellectual or artistic love.

Contrary to myth, love is not inexplicable or beyond understanding. Love can be exactly defined and clearly understood.

Romantic love integrates the mind and body of a man and a woman. That integration includes the emotional/intellectual development of values between that man and woman. Such a complex relationship requires planned, rational thought by each partner.

Yet romantic love is often dismissed as blind, mindless, irrational, immature, transitory, or impractical. But the opposite is true. And similar false notions have led to the misunderstanding of words such as 'romantic', 'romanticism', and the 'Romantic era'.

How did those false notions begin? 'Romantic' and its related words originally implied freedom, individuality, and rational ideals based on integrated honesty; not irrational whims based on mystical illusions. But over the years, the concept of romanticism became inverted by the mystics (and more recently the media) and falsely associated with the irrationalists and the sentimentalists of the 19th Century Romantic Period.

Romantic love involves an emotional, intellectual, and sexual involvement with another person. Romantic love offers the deepest of all happiness and the greatest of all pleasures. But as with all major values, romantic love is not automatic. Romantic love must be earned through rational thought and planned effort. And then, that love must

---

[106] Philosopher Blaze Pascal, www.centralpc.org/sermons/2003/s030427.htm

be maintained and expanded through constant honest effort -- through constant discipline, thought, and control.

So the reason for the negativity in previous discussions was to break the beliefs many hold about relationships, in preparation for this section, which highlights the reason why Freedom Technology regards and promotes the concepts of Fascinating Relationships according to Universal Truths. Get ready for it.

Here's a question which you may not have been prepared for: "Will there be sex in heaven (or, as we now know it, the E5)?"

It is a question not many have allowed themselves to wonder, even though the question bears asking.

The Union That We Crave

To understand the importance of the question, you have to recognize the ache that seems to be met only through sexual union. When God created Eve, as you will recall, He took her straight from Adam's side. None of us have fully recovered from the surgery. There is an aloneness, an incompleteness that we experience every day of our lives.

How often do you feel deeply and truly known? Is there another soul to whom a simple glance is all that is necessary to communicate depth of understanding? This is our inconsolable longing — to know and to be known.

It is our deepest ache, which we feel to be healed only in our union with another - even physically. There is an incompleteness until our bodies are joined together.

But let us take a closer look. What are we looking for in the opposite sex?

The Beloved in Song of Songs (a book in the Bible) captures something of what the heart of a woman is seeking. There is an emptiness in the woman that only her man can fill. Is it not physically true?

But it is more than just physically true. Our bodies are an outward sign of an inward reality.

So, too, the woman completes her man in a uniquely beautiful way.

"Come to me", she says, "and let your strength be fully expressed in the garden of my beauty".

Is this not the invitation that stirs a man's heart?

These are the qualities of the Beloved that captivate her Lover in the Song. He says,

"How beautiful you are, my darling!
Oh, how beautiful!
Your eyes behind your veil are doves . . .
Your lips are like a scarlet ribbon, your mouth is lovely ...

Your two breasts are like two fawns,
like twin fawns of a gazelle that browse among the lilies."[107]

There is no union on earth like the consummation of the love between a man and a woman. No other connection reaches as deeply as this oneness was meant to; no other passion is nearly so intense.

People do not jump off bridges because they lost a grandparent. If their friend makes another friend, they do not shoot them both. No one has ruined home and career for a rendezvous at the library. Troy did not go down in flames because somebody lost a pet.

The passion that spousal love evokes is instinctive, irrational, intense and dare we say, immortal. As the Song says,

"Love is as strong as death,
its jealousy unyielding as the grave.
It burns like a blazing fire,
like a mighty flame.
Many waters cannot quench love,
rivers cannot wash it away."[108]

Small wonder that many people experience sexual passion as their highest transcendence on this earth. This love surpasses all others as the source of the world's most beautiful poetry, art, and music.

Lovers reach for the stars to find words fitting enough to express what the beloved means to them and still feel those words fall short. Granted, much of it is hyperbole and exaggeration, expressing more the dream than the reality. But that is precisely our point. It is not merely hormones and sex drives projected outward. It is not merely our natural instinct. It is a clue to a deeper reality, a reach for something that *does* exist.

This exotic intimacy was given to us as a picture of something else, something truly out of this world.

Our Love Affair with God

After creating this stunning portrait of a total union, the man and woman becoming one, God turns the Universe on its head when He tells us that *this is what He is seeking with us!*

In fact, Paul (in the Bible) says it is why God created gender and sexuality and marriage — to serve as a living metaphor or example. He quotes Genesis, and then takes it to the highest degree:

"For this reason a man will leave his father and mother and be united to his wife, and the two will become one flesh. This is a profound mystery — but I am talking about Christ and the church".[109]

---

[107] Song of Songs 4:1, 3, 5 NIV
[108] Song of Songs 8:6-7 NIV
[109] Ephesians 5:31-32 NIV

Yes, go and read it – it is what the Bible says about sex! It is an example of the relationship with God. A profound mystery indeed. All the breathtaking things in life are deep.

The Cross is a great mystery, but we are helped in understanding it by looking back into the Old Testament and finding there the pattern of the sacrificial lamb. Those early believers did not understand the full meaning of what they were doing, but once Christ came, the whole period of ritual sacrifice was seen in a new light, and in turn gave a richer depth to our understanding of the Cross.

We must do the same with this stunning passage - we must look back and see the Bible for what it is — the greatest romance ever written. God creates mankind for intimacy with himself, as His beloved.

We see it right at the start, when He gives us the highest freedom of all — the freedom to reject him. The reason is obvious: love is possible only when it is freely chosen. True love is never constrained or forced; our hearts cannot be taken by force.

So God sets out to woo his beloved and make her His queen:

"I gave you my solemn oath and entered into a covenant with you, declares the Sovereign Lord, and you became Mine . . . I dressed you in fine linen and covered you with costly garments. I adorned you with jewelry. . . You became very beautiful and rose to be a queen. And your fame spread among the nations on account of your beauty, because the splendor I had given you made your beauty perfect." [110]

"In that day", declares the LORD, "you will call me 'my husband'; you will no longer call me 'my master'." [111]

'That day' comes when Jesus appears on the scene and announces himself as the Bridegroom. [112]

And when He says to us, "I am going there to prepare a place for you. And if I go and prepare a place for you, I will come back and take you to be with me that you also may be where I am", he is making his proposal. [113]

In the culture of the day, these are the very words a young man would say to his fiancée. Once the suitor secured the hand of his bride, he would return to his father's house and build the additional room that would be their bridal suite. (Couples moved into the home of the groom's parents.)

---

[110] Ezekiel 16.8, 10-11, 13-14 NIV
[111] Hosea 3:6-7, 14, 16 NIV
[112] Matthew 9:15
[113] John 14:2-3 NIV

It was 'preparing a place for her'. When all was ready, he would come for her and take her to be with him, so that where he is, she would also be.

We, the beloved, have become betrothed (engaged, married) to the Bridegroom. And will be taken by Him into the E5.

John the Baptist said, "The bride belongs to the bridegroom. The friend who attends the bridegroom waits and listens for him, and is full of joy when he hears the bridegroom's voice."[114]

We are in the time of waiting for the Bridegroom to return.

By the end of the love story in Revelation 22, the church is practically panting for the return of Christ:

"The Spirit and Bride say, "Come!" And let him who hears say "Come!" Whoever is thirsty, let him come; and whoever wishes, let him take the free gift of the water of life ... He who testifies to these things says, "Yes, I am coming soon! Amen. Come Lord Jesus."[115]

Notice that it is the bride who is panting. How does a bride pant? As if for a lover who has long been away. She pants like the Beloved in Song of Songs "Come, my lover, let us go to the countryside . . . There I will give you my love."[116] We are waiting for our Love to come and take us to His home!

Augustine declared, "The whole life of the good Christian is a holy longing. What you desire ardently, as yet you do not see . . . By withholding of the vision, God extends the longing, through longing he extends the soul, by extending He makes room in it".

So, said Augustine, "let us long because we are to be filled . . . that is our life, to be exercised by longing."

And when The Bridegroom of our souls comes, what then?

The Consummation of the Affair

What is worship, after all?

The older Christian wedding vows contained these amazing words: "With my body, I thee worship."

Maybe our forefathers were not so prudish after all. Maybe they understood sex far better than we do. To give yourself over to another, passionately and nakedly, to adore that person body, soul, and spirit — we know there is something special, even sacramental or divine about sex. It requires trust and abandonment, guided by a wholehearted devotion. What else can this be but worship? After all, God employs explicitly sexual language to describe faithfulness (and unfaithfulness) to him.

---

[114] John 3:29 NIV
[115] Revelation 22:17, 20 NIV
[116] Song of Songs 7:11-12 NIV

For us creatures of the flesh, sexual intimacy is the closest parallel we have to real worship. Even the world knows this. Why else would sexual ecstasy become the number one rival to communion with God? The best impostors succeed because they are nearly indistinguishable from what they are trying to imitate. We worship sex because we do not know how to worship God. But we will.

Peter Kreeft writes: "This spiritual intercourse with God is the ecstasy hinted at in all earthly intercourse, physical or spiritual.

"It is the ultimate reason why sexual passion is so strong, so different from other passions, so heavy with suggestions of profound meanings that just elude our grasp."[117]

Do not let your possibly disappointing experiences cloud your understanding of this. We have grown cynical, as a society, about whether intimacy is really possible. To the degree that we have abandoned soul-oneness, we have sought out merely sex, physical sex, to ease the pain. The full union is no longer there, the orgasm comes incomplete, its heart has been taken away. Many have been deeply hurt.

Sometimes, we must learn from what we have not known; let it teach us what ought to be. God's design was that the two shall become one flesh. The physical oneness was meant to be the expression of a total inter-weaving of being. Is it any wonder that we crave this?

Our alienation is removed, if only for a moment and in the paradox of love, we are at the same time known and taken beyond ourselves.

In *The Mystery of Marriage*, Mike Mason asserts: "For many people, certainly, sex is the most powerful and moving experience that life has to offer, and more overwhelmingly holy than anything that happens in church.

"For great masses of people, sex is the one force which can actually tip men and women completely off their accustomed centers of gravity and lift them, however briefly, right out of themselves."

As Allender says, our hearts live for "an experience of worship that fills our beings with joy that is so deeply in awe of the other that we are barely aware of ourselves."[118]

Many people have a hard time conceiving of this kind of intimacy with God. For their entire lives they have related to Him in a distant, though reverent way. Most church worship services are not anything like our wedding nights.

Men in particular have a hard time relating to the bridal imagery used in Scripture. Do we take on femininity to relate to God? What does it mean to 'know' God as our Lover?

---

[117] Quoted in *The Journey of Desire* by John Eldridge, Nelson Books, 2000
[118] Quoted in *The Mystery of Marriage* by Mike Mason, Multnomah, 2001

The Beauty and Strength of God

It is a mystery almost too great to mention, but God is the expression of the very thing we seek in each other. Do we not bear God's image? Are we not a living portrait of God? Of course we are, and in a most surprising place — in our gender.

> "So God created man in his own image, in the image of God he created him, male and female he created them."[119]

Follow us closely now. Gender — masculinity and femininity — is how we bear the image of God.

"I thought that there was only one kind of soul," said a shocked friend; "And God sort of poured those souls into male or female bodies."

Many people believe something very similar. But it contradicts the Word of God. We bear his image as men and women. The text is clear; it is as a man or as a woman that the image is bestowed.

God wanted to show the world something of His strength. Is He not a great warrior? Has He not performed the daring rescue of his beloved? And this is why He gave us the sculpture that is man. Men bear the image of God in their dangerous, yet inviting strength.

Women, too, bear the image of God, but in a far different way. Is not God a being of great mystery and beauty? Is there not something tender and alluring about the essence of the Divine? And this is why He gave us the sculpture that is woman.

"My wife's body is more fascinating than a flower, shier than any animal, and more breathtaking than a thousand sunsets. To me her body is the most awesome thing in creation. Trying to look at her, just trying to take in her wild, glorious beauty . . . I catch a glimpse of what it means that men and women have been made in the image of God. If even the image is this dazzling, what must the Original be like?"[120]

What, indeed. God is the source of all masculine power; God is also the fountain of all feminine allure. Come to think of it, He is the wellspring of everything that has ever romanced your heart: The thundering strength of a waterfall, the delicacy of a flower, the stirring capacity of music, the richness of wine.

The masculine and the feminine that fill all creation come from the same heart. What we have sought, what we have tasted in part with our earthly lovers, we will come face-to-face with in our True Love.

The incompleteness that we seek to relieve in the deep embrace of our earthly love is never fully healed. The union does not last, whatever the poets, authors and pop artists may say. Morning comes and we have got to get out of bed and off to our day, incomplete once more.

---

[119] Genesis 1:17 NIV
[120] Quoted in *The Mystery of Marriage* by Mike Mason, Multnomah, 2001

But oh, to have it healed forever, to drink deeply from that fount of which we have had only a sip, to dive into that sea in which we have only waded.

And so a man like Charles Wesley can pen these words: "Jesus, Lover of my soul, let me to thy bosom fly".

While Catherine of Siena can pray: "O fire surpassing every fire because you alone are the fire that burns without consuming . . . Yet your consuming does not distress the soul but fattens her with insatiable love."

The French mystic Madame Guyon can write: "I slept not all night, because Thy love, O my God, flowed in me like delicious oil, and burned as a fire ... I love God far more than the most affectionate lover among men loves his earthly attachment."[121]

And at the same time a monk, St. John of the Cross can say: "I abandoned and forgot myself, laying my face on my Beloved, all things ceased; I went out from myself leaving my cares forgotten among the lilies."

Where else are we told about oil and lilies? In Song of Songs.

Is there sex in heaven? It would be better to ask, "Is there worship in heaven?"

It is a manifestation of the humility of God that He creates a kingdom so rich in love that He should not be our all; but that others should be precious to us as well. Even in Eden, before the Fall, while Adam walked in Paradise with his God, even then God said, "It is not good for the man to be alone".[122] He gives to us the joy of community, of family and friends to share in the Sacred Romance.

Is it not the nature of true love — to be generous in love?

This is something of the reason that married couples long to have children; they want others to share in their happiness. The embrace of lovers does not stay confined to the lovers; rather, it builds a home, it fills a household. And so our longing for intimacy reaches beyond our 'one and only'. We come to discover that others mean so very much to us.

There is no joy like the joy of reunion because there is no sorrow like the sorrow of separation. To lose those we love and wonder if we shall ever see them again — this is our deepest grief.

What is vital for us to grasp is this: The life we now have as the persons we now are, will continue in the Universe that is to come. By all means we will know each other's name – not if but when we see each other in God's great kingdom. We will hold each other's hands, and far better than that. The naked intimacy, the real knowing that we enjoy with God, we shall enjoy with each other.

---

[121] www.housechurch.org/spirituality/guyon_autobio1.html
[122] Genesis 2:18 NIV

George MacDonald wrote, "I think we shall be able to pass into and through each other's very souls as we please, knowing each other's thought and being, along with our own, and so being like God."[123]

Brent calls it 'multiple intimacy without promiscuity'. It is what the ancients meant by 'the communion of saints'.[124]

All of the joy that awaits us in the sea of God's love will be multiplied over and over as we share with each other in the Grand Affair. The setting for this will be a great party, the wedding feast of the Lamb.

Now, you have to get the images of the typical church receptions entirely out of your mind — folks milling around in the church gym, holding Styrofoam cups of non-alcoholic drinks, wondering what to do with themselves.

You have got to picture an Italian wedding or, better, a Jewish wedding. They roll up the rugs and push back the furniture. There is dancing:

"Then maidens will dance and be glad, young men and old as well"[125]

There is feasting:

"On this mountain the LORD Almighty will prepare a feast of rich food for all peoples"[126]

Can you imagine what kind of cook God must be?

And there is drinking — the feast God says he is preparing includes:

"a banquet of aged wine — the best of meats and the finest of wines."

In fact, at his Last Supper our Bridegroom said He will not drink of "the fruit of the vine until the kingdom of God comes." [127]

Then he'll pop a cork, and the Party will begin.

As you make love, remember it is rehearsal for the Grand Affair!

The Meaning of Freedom

No matter how much one puts into establishing freedom by the bullet or even by the ballot, it simply cannot be achieved in this world. This is the great utopian delusion which lies at the heart of all humanistic illuminism.

While one does not want to see dictatorships at work in the world, the fact is that true human freedom is determined neither by

---

[123] www.johannesen.com/HopeoftheGospelComplete.htm
[124] As quoted in *The Journey of Desire* by John Eldridge, Nelson Books, 2000
[125] Jeremiah 3:13 NIV
[126] Isaiah 25:6 NIV
[127] Luke 22:18 NIV

governments nor by revolutions. One can be emancipated from the worst political dictator and yet still fail to be free. Conversely, one can be a captive in the world's darkest dungeon and yet be totally at liberty.

How is that possible?

Because true freedom consists not in physical liberty, but in spiritual liberty.

Such liberty comes only through knowing the truth and acting upon it. There is no greater liberating force than that; and it has one source only - in Jesus Christ, the Son of God, the symbol of materialization from the E5 to the E4 and back.

This may come as a surprise, considering our extremely negative view of religion in previous chapters. However, the views expressed in previous chapters were necessary so that you can accept that we say this without the influence of myths and other fables.

Believing in the message of Jesus Christ is the only action which brings liberty. As He said: "You shall know the truth, and the truth shall make you free"[128]

Christ's public ministry was dedicated to the total liberation of human beings, as He announced when He began to preach: "[God] has anointed me...to proclaim liberty to the captives." [129]

Just what was the 'liberty' which Christ proclaimed? Was Jesus a political activist, or was he a good Communist, as was claimed by Fidel Castro? Did Jesus offer liberty from cruel human tyrants? From famine? From poverty?

Not at all. It was freedom from the state of bondage to sin (the negative force) in which all human beings find themselves,[130] freedom from domination by the fallen angel Satan,[131] and freedom from every aspect of death.[132] That is the kind of freedom which is offered by Christ - which lasts not only in this life, but for all eternity (the E5).

This is a truly revolutionary freedom - infinitely transcending anything which governments or guerrilla leaders can offer.

Jesus' Secret Message

The following is adapted from an essay by Tracey Alexander, quoted in Neo-Tech.[133]

In order to understand the New Testament and Jesus' message one must first know the distinction between the conscious mind and the bicameral mind. With that knowledge Jesus' message becomes clear.

---

[128] John 8:32
[129] Luke 4:18
[130] John 8:34-36, 41-44
[131] 1 John 3:8; Mark 3:27
[132] Hebrews 2:14-15
[133] www.neo-tech.com/

This new way of thinking involves an understanding of the right hemisphere of the brain vs. the left hemisphere. Bicameral man used both sides but in a different way than we do today. The right hemisphere is our survival mechanism...automatic reactions to sights, sounds and emotions. Faced with dangerous situations one must react quickly and automatically...totally immersed in the here and now. Also for survival skills one must be able to recognize the overall picture, to grasp the larger perspective. This function can be seen as necessary for survival in early man when out hunting and being able to find his way home...and is responsible for some of our most creative insights. It is the function of putting all the pieces together in an overall larger picture.

However our right hemisphere has a major flaw as far as consciousness is concerned. And that is, it has no judgmental ability. Bicameral man lived by his natural, highly intelligent animal mind. And the animal mind has no concept of justice, fairness, or compassion. Therefore bicameral man lived by social 'codes of conduct' necessary for people to live harmoniously in a society. Moses' Ten Commandments is an example of a 'code of conduct' given by an authority figure for the Hebrew nation to follow. Notice that all ten commands relate to objective behavior...there is no inner reason given as to why these commands are necessary. Even though to us it is self evident why these commands are valid, it was not until the later prophets and especially with Jesus that the inner reasons for this behavior was known.

The bicameral man lacked introspection and could not know for himself what was moral or immoral. This explains many of the mysteries of the Old Testament when a tribe favored by God would conquer another tribe, kill the men, women and children and take all of their goods, cattle, sheep, etc. There was no concept of justice, compassion, or wrong-doing on their part. When we read these stories today, we cannot reconcile that kind of behavior with God's condolence. In the light of the bicameral mind, however, these actions become clear. There is no blame.

The bicameral man felt emotions strongly, just as we see in nature when a mother lion fiercely protects her young.

A major factor in becoming conscious and understanding Jesus' ministry is introspection. Not just feeling emotions as all animals do and reacting automatically to those emotions but understanding emotions. Without 'understanding' emotions no concept of justice or compassion could emerge. The interaction of the feeling right hemisphere with the rational, objective left hemisphere allows consciousness to emerge.

Just what is consciousness? One chief factor is the ability to be objective, to put aside your emotions, and weigh a situation honestly...a feature bicameral man could not do. With this ability to be objective a man can think in terms of the past and the future, not just in the present, in the here and now, as the right hemisphere does. With that ability a man can think in terms of changing his behavior – Jesus' emphasis on forgiveness and compassion.

The world we live in is a reflection of who we are inwardly as individuals. Our businesses, our schools, our governments are all run by individuals and the laws and traditions that we believe in or allow to exist determine our outer conditions. It is only as we understand ourselves, what is good for us and what is bad for us, that we can we take the right actions for a fulfilled life. And we also extend that same privilege to others.

That introspection, that getting in touch with and understanding our own emotions, leads to the conscious awareness of what is moral, good and right. That process lies at the heart of Jesus' message. Through this route a surprise emerges. Jesus' call to the weary, the suffering, and the lonely was a constant theme throughout his ministry. Those who are unhappy in some way are the most likely to introspect. Also 'following His example' with the difficult trials he had to face is a way toward introspection, a major route to consciousness and the knowledge and wisdom of the 'Kingdom of God'.

Consciousness was developed about three thousand years ago. As societies became more and more complex, the bicameral mind became inadequate to cope. This new way of thinking coincides roughly with the rule of King David in the Old Testament. Moses lived in the thirteenth century B.C. which puts Abraham, the father of the Hebrew nation, even earlier. Historically then the early books of the Bible are stories of bicameral men. Those who lived by codes of conduct handed down to them by authority figures.

The Old Testament prophets give a vivid picture of the awakening of consciousness in man with the culmination in Jesus' ministry.

There are two major stages to consciousness, to becoming aware. The first stage has to do with ethics and moral behavior. And this requires complete honesty.

In following Jesus' example, He said you must die and be reborn. This is a metaphor, of course, but you must die to the old ways of thinking which keep you locked in a life of slavery to traditions. Through introspection and examination you come to realize that contrary to church doctrines and religious beliefs you must act in a way that supports the Immutable Laws of Nature, as opposed to man-made laws.

The second major stage to consciousness is to become your own authority. This was clearly evident with Jesus who spoke with authority...and we are supposed to follow His example. In speaking with authority Jesus completely amazed the people because no religious leader of the time spoke in such a manner. Jesus and his disciples broke many of the religious laws of his time. When confronted by the Pharisees, Jesus said that laws were made for man, not man for the laws.

Once a person is conscious of ethical and honest behavior and the inner and psychological reasons why that behavior is essential to his and others' happiness, then he is ready to become his own authority. However, a person must start living a self directed life to build the confidence needed to break through to the second stage...to become his own authority.

That is why Jesus spoke in metaphors and parables to the crowds. You cannot make a huge leap in consciousness until the groundwork is first laid. Developing consciousness and becoming your own authority is clearly Jesus' message. And in order to be your own authority you must break with all authorities, including the authority of man-made religions.

With a fully conscious mind, we are ready to step into what Jesus called 'The Kingdom of God'.[134]

Why the Emphasis on the Biblical World View?

It is our aim and hope that you will be empowered to achieve a bigger view of life than the average, leading to true happiness. A way of life, a path that leads to enlightenment and fulfillment, heart-peace, satisfaction, joy, life to the full, fully alive and vibrant, becoming all you were meant to be, recognizing the powers within and exercising them fully, discovering your true purpose in life; having understanding of life's questions of meaning, morality and destiny.

Science Reveals the Ultimate Truth

Pursuit of truth is, and must remain, the driving force behind scientific endeavor. The more accurate the assessment of the environment by an individual, the more appropriate and harmonious that mind is with the nuances of the changing environment i.e. the more in-touch with reality that person is.

An underlying wisdom and unity pervade the Universe, life, and the human mind. Scientists exposed this discovery in their quest to uncover the ultimate nature of reality.

---

[134] Adapted from an essay by Tracey Alexander, quoted in Neo-Tech

And this wisdom is reflected in the pages of the Bible. Wisdom which is often hidden in parables and other secret messages reserved only for those with the required discipline and hunger to search out the real meanings. Religion is thus the lazy option, where interpretations are made by an elite clergy and spoon-fed to an indolent, lethargic congregation. These teachings are at best hollow and meaningless, at worst intentionally misleading.

The Biblical World View is the only world view which provides a succinct meaning of life, and a profound purpose for our existence. The logic of that purpose, coupled with the Immutable Laws of Nature surpasses that of any other competing idea or philosophy.

If you can grasp this integrative principle, then you will have a useful filter through which information can be sorted and choices made.

You will have the road map to a life of personal freedom; relationship success; glowing health, longevity and weight management; sufficient income; and metaphysical balance.

This manual thus provides the key to a new life for you, based on knowledge and control. The approach is simply an extrapolation of the logic and understanding you already possess, but may not have pieced together into the giant jigsaw puzzle of life.

Remember this wonderful irony: readers who reap the greatest benefit from *Fresh Wisdom* encounter passages about which they initially disagree, even bitterly disagree. Yet, as they continue reading, negative impressions fade as long-suppressed facts combined with brand new integrations increasingly enrich their lives with power, wealth, health and romance.

Remember that we are not trying to persuade you of any political, religious, ideological or philosophical position. We hold no such positions, since we apply only the Immutable Laws of Nature.

We hope that this chapter has opened your eyes to the previously suppressed power of the Biblical World View. This understanding is important as we progress to the next exciting topic, which is Reaching Your Own Personal Omega Point.

If ultimate reality consists of elementary particles, and if everything that has happened is in some sense determined by some great law that governed events at the beginning of the Big Bang, then the search for the final theory is not just a game that Particle Physicists play but a quest of immense importance to humanity.

If an Initiator exists and has revealed something of His nature to humankind, then the interaction of Initiator and the whole of creation is not just the most complex of subjects, but by far the most important.

17. Your Personal Omega Point

We are nearing the end of this manual, but we are also nearing the start of a completely new life. You may not even be aware of how much your way of thinking has already changed since commencing this journey.

Here is a reminder of the quote that started this entire manual. It was Marianne Williamson, who said this:

"Our deepest fear is not that we are inadequate. Our deepest fear is that we are powerful beyond measure. It is our light, not our darkness, that most frightens us.

We ask ourselves, "Who am I to be brilliant, gorgeous, talented and fabulous?"

Actually, who are you not to be? You are a child of God. Your playing small does not serve the world. There is nothing enlightened about shrinking so that other people will not feel insecure around you. We were born to manifest the glory of God that is within us. And as we let our own light shine, we unconsciously give other people permission to do the same.

As we are liberated from our own fear, our presence automatically liberates others." -- Marianne Williamson (often incorrectly stated as a quote from Nelson Mandela).[135]

We have reached the stage where we tie all the various "Aha!" experiences we have enjoyed together, into a very powerful principle, by answering the question: "Why am I here?" In answering this question you will have reached your personal Omega Point, and if we can help you to do so your life will dramatically, almost magically rocket-propel itself from one of "playing small" to one that is "powerful beyond measure".

Lofty words, we agree. And yet, the process is simple and results are nothing short of spectacular. It does take some mental discipline, thought and control, but if you have made it thus far, the rest should be a breeze.

What is The Omega Point?

The Omega point is a term originally coined by Pierre Teilhard de Chardin[136] to describe the aim towards which consciousness evolves. Frank J. Tipler[137], also a supporter of the Omega point, has proposed that it is possible for intelligent beings to process and store an infinite

---

[135] http://skdesigns.com/internet/articles/quotes/williamson.html
[136] http://en.wikipedia.org/wiki/Omega_point
[137] www.aleph.se/Trans/Global/Omega/

amount of information in the Universe, if certain conditions are fulfilled.

In *Fresh Wisdom*, we use the term to mean the *point of ultimate understanding*, since the Greek 'omega' (as in alpha and omega) refers to the pinnacle of ultimate understanding. It is the definitive "Aha!" experience, when the purpose of life suddenly becomes clear.

According to many futurists, there is a sheath of information technology covering the planet, and this Technosphere is the material basis of the now awakening Noosphere - earth's mental envelope or field. The word Noosphere derives from the Greek "noos", or "nous", and means mind, while "sphere", or "spheria," means globe. It is therefore the globe of thought, and includes all knowledge of collective humanity. This is a similar paradigm to Carl Jung's *collective unconscious*.

If you are interested in reading more about this Technosphere and man's awakening collective consciousness, see *Awakening to the Omega Point: Chardin and the Noosphere*.[138] However, before you read the article, it is important that you understand our view on this Noosphere. We certainly agree that the concept of global consciousness exists; however reaching your personal Omega Point is the ability *to break away* from this mentally limiting bubble. By its very definition, the Noosphere described in the above-mentioned article is not a positive force, but the worst form of enslavement humankind could ever be subjected to.

In short, reaching your personal Omega Point, as described in *Fresh Wisdom*, requires the ability to:

- Accept the current state of your life, your environment, the planet, the Universe, your past, your beliefs and your (current) future aspirations;
- Identify the con's in that image;
- Trash those con's as worthless (or step outside of the bubble – the Noosphere);
- Define a new purpose, free of the limiting beliefs which previously held you back, and in so doing reach your Personal Omega Point.

In essence, reaching your personal Omega Point answers the question "Why am I here?" and this cannot be achieved while held captive by limiting beliefs.

Can you see now why we had to spend so much time identifying the erroneous beliefs early in earlier chapters? We had to encourage you to reach the point where you could objectively analyze everything you have previously accepted as absolute reality, so that you

---

[138] http://omegapoint.org/modules/news/article.php?storyid=10

can dump the faulty lines of code in the program currently running in your mind. We are encouraging you to remove yourself from the destructive Noosphere.

Incidentally, in the next chapter we will discuss a process called *The Ten Second Miracle*, whereby in 10 seconds, you can do exactly that – dump the faulty lines of code. But once again, we are getting ahead of ourselves.

Omega Point Definition

Here is a succinct definition of the Omega Point. Note that the brevity of the definition of a concept that has Universal implications automatically precludes covering all aspects of the concept.

> *The Omega Point is the peak of a pyramid of ultimate understanding of the Universe and man's purpose in that Universe at that point in time, without the influence of fables and traditions.*

We must stress the phrase 'at that point in time'. It is impossible for any human to possess and store all known knowledge. Therefore the Omega Point can be reached more than once during a lifetime, as your knowledge and understanding grows exponentially. It goes without saying, though, that reaching your first Omega Point is a mind-blowing, life-altering experience.

Let us try to explain this diagrammatically.

The Pinnacle of Understanding

During your *Fresh Wisdom* journey thus far, you may have experienced many "Aha!" moments. If you remember back to the first chapter (with the picture of the old and young woman), we explained that each "Aha!" experience is a paradigm shift – a new world view, or a new way of receiving, filtering and processing information based on the presence or otherwise of preconditions. We encourage you to read that short chapter on page 16 again if you need a refresher on conditioning – it is important groundwork to understand the principles we are about to discuss.

Each of those "Aha!" experiences can be described as a mini-triangle of learning, leading towards The Omega Point.

Imagine a pyramid made up of a set of smaller pyramids and other tightly-fitting geometric shapes. Each shape within the pyramid is crucial for a stable pyramid – remove one, or change its shape, and the entire pyramid collapses.

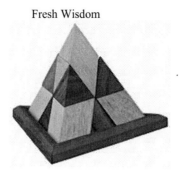

The Triangular Theory of Consciousness

This same concept can be applied to the human brain.

From extensive studies in hospitals relating to mindsets and rates of recovery (led by Dr Ian Weinberg,[139]) it was discovered that specific areas in the brain appear to be programmed for receptivity of the particular environmental entity [what appears in *your* life]. Each successively higher group represents a more specific representation of what that mind perceives; thus representing in the brain a microcosm of the entire environment.

As an example: viewing a tree creates an impression in the mind of its existence. If not viewed through a distorting lens, it is an accurate representation. Therefore the tree 'exists' in the mind.

This principle applies to all of life. Correct perception leads to perfect understanding. There exists a process of *integration* in the brain.

Imagine a set of ten triangles along a base line: the apex of each representing the whole.

Now imagine three triangles above the lower ten, each in turn being a summation of the triangles below. The apexes of each of these three triangles are now summed up in one triangle above the three, representing the summation of the three and thus the final summation of the original ten.

This represents the process of 'integrating' or 'nodal representation'.

The final integration at the node of the top triangle represents Omega Point or the final integration node.

An even closer representation is one in three dimensions, where the triangles are cones.

So, the *best* model is one where there are many cones, close fitted, supporting a pyramid of similar ones. This represents taking into account *all* the factors impacting an environment, giving a truer

---

[139] '*Quantum-determinism – an Integrative Model of Holistic Consciousness*' by Dr Ian Weinberg. Published in *Quantum Leap*, Sygma Books, 1998

summation. The node of each lower order being represented in the higher, focusing on the final node: Omega Point.

The *worst* model is a series of unrelated cones attempting to support others. Elements which do not fit or do not match with a particular bias are filtered out, rejected, leaving a very poor representation of the environment.

This is typical of people who are strongly held by tradition or other people's opinions and who are not able to comfortably integrate new information, since it does not coincide with preconceived frameworks.

But, the results of the medical studies indicated that biases affect perception, distorting reality.

There are basically 3 types of mindset, each having their own limitations or freedoms:

1. **No Filters**: This is a mindset that can be represented by a whole series of perfectly formed cones supporting ever higher levels of condensed information cones; leading ultimately to a pinnacle cone representing Omega Point or perfect understanding.

   When reviewing new information, the mindset is not influenced by predetermined views, but perceives the matter without trying to make it fit preconceived ideas.

   This is the gold standard, with no bias when interpreting new information. This type holds a true reflection of the external environment and is able to deal in a balanced manner with the external changing environment.

2. **Tall Cones**: This type can be represented by a base of tall cones that cannot support ever-increasing levels of other cones, since they do not contact the bases of higher levels, causing them to fall in between the base cones, forming a disjointed pattern.

   Thus it represents a mind that is not integrated. Sensed information is distorted to fit or it is deleted completely, not allowing the mind to form a true perspective of the world.

   It manifests in insecurity and driven personalities. When forced out of the comfort zone of islands this person becomes insecure; momentarily loses their way resulting in a feeling of temporary purposelessness which also results (according to the studies this was based on) an impairment of immune function. Mind states thus *do* affect states of health.

3. **Excessive Filters**: This type of mind map consists of many small un-integrated islands, and is not able to support any higher levels. It has difficulty in making any sense of the environment.

In summary, the more accurate the assessment of the environment by an individual, the more appropriate and harmonious that mind is with the nuances of the changing environment.

In this situation of no filters, success of one's actions is guaranteed - reinforcing further positive feedback. The immune system is enhanced and the individual experiences a vital existence for a long period.

This would indicate a person who sought truth at any cost to their own discomfort. In other words, the more regularly an individual goes outside their comfort zones, the more in-touch with *reality* that person is.

Another person, when forced out of the comfort zone of islands, refuses to accept, rejects, becomes insecure, and momentarily loses their way, temporary purposelessness, impairment of immune function.

In conclusion, if an individual can correctly view their external environment and they are on an upward path of self-actualization and self-transcendence, they *are* able to reach their personal Omega Point.

This principle applies to all of life. Correct perception leads to perfect understanding.

~~~

Side Note: It should come as no surprise then that pyramids have long been the favorite symbol of secret societies, representing the pinnacle of understanding.

Readers may be familiar with the symbol on the reverse of the US $1 bill, showing an all-seeing eye atop an incomplete pyramid.

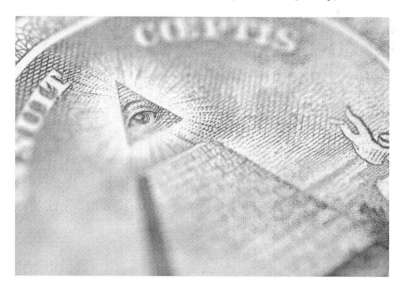

Space and time limitations preclude us from explaining the symbolism behind this diagram – if you are interested in reading more, see *The All Seeing Eye.*[140]

Maslow's Hierarchy of Needs

At this point it is important to discuss Maslow's Hierarchy of Needs[141], because if your basic needs are not met, it is unlikely you will achieve the Omega Point.

Maslow posited a hierarchy of human needs based on two groupings: Deficiency Needs and Growth Needs.

Within the Deficiency Needs, each lower need must be met before moving to the next higher level. Once each of these needs has been satisfied, if at some future time a deficiency is detected, the individual will act to remove the deficiency.

The first Deficiency Needs consist of four levels:
1. Physiological: hunger, thirst, bodily comforts, etc.;
2. Safety and Security: avoiding danger;
3. Belongingness and Love: affiliate with others, be accepted; and
4. Esteem: to achieve, be competent, gain approval and recognition.

An individual is ready to act upon the Growth Needs only when the Deficiency Needs are met. In other words, it is unlikely you will be concerned about the beauty of your garden if you are constantly hungry. Once the basic needs are met, that individual can move on to the higher levels.

There are two levels of Growth Needs:
5. Cognitive: to know, to understand, and explore;
6. Aesthetic: symmetry, order, and beauty.

Maslow then identified further Growth Needs:
7. Self-Actualization: to find self-fulfillment and realizing of one's full potential;
8. Self-Transcendence: to connect to something beyond the ego or to help others find self-fulfillment and realize their potential.

Maslow described Self-Actualization as follows: A musician must make music, the artist must paint, a poet must write, if he is to be ultimately at peace with himself. What a man can be, he must be.

Maslow writes of self-actualizing people that:
- They embrace the facts and realities of the world (including themselves) rather than denying or avoiding them.
- They are spontaneous in their ideas and actions.
- They are creative.

---

[140] www.conspiracyarchive.com/NWO/All_Seeing_Eye.htm
[141] http://en.wikipedia.org/wiki/Maslow's_hierarchy_of_needs

- They are interested in solving problems; this often includes the problems of others. Solving these problems is often a key focus in their lives.
- They feel a closeness to other people, and generally appreciate life.
- They have a system of morality that is fully internalized and independent of external authority.
- They judge others without prejudice, in a way that can be termed objective.

Sounds like Maslow was describing a *Fresh Thinker*, does it not?

Maslow's basic position is that as one becomes more self-actualized and self-transcendent, one develops wisdom and automatically knows how to cope in a wide variety of situations. Maslow's ultimate conclusion is that the highest levels of self-actualization are transcendent in their nature. This may be one of his most important contributions to the study of human behavior and motivation.

Maslow's hierarchy can be used to describe the kinds of information that individual's seek at different levels.

Coping Information – is sought by individuals at the lowest level who need methods and answers in order to meet their most basic needs of sustaining life.

Helping Information – is sought by individuals wanting to meet their needs in a quicker manner, for example, improving the process of acquiring food. Individuals at the coping level need helping information.

Enlightening Information – is sought by individuals wanting to belong within a functioning, relatively safe environment. Quite often this can be found in books or other materials on relationship development.

Empowering Information - is sought by people at the esteem level. They are looking for information on how their ego can be developed.

Edifying Information – is sought by individuals wanting to connect to something beyond themselves, or assisting others in enlightening themselves.

Once again, unless you believe your Cognitive and Aesthetic Needs have been met, or are in the process of being met, it is unlikely that achieving your personal Omega Point is just around the corner. *Fresh Wisdom* assists in providing the required Enlightening, Empowering and Edifying Information to achieve your personal Omega Point.

This is a further reason *Fresh Wisdom* covers the 5 Essential Pillars of Fulfilled Living: unless you achieve full understanding (without the influence of fables and traditions) in each one of the 5 Pillars, your pyramid is likely to be unstable.

A little later we will cover the 5 Pillars again, in relation to The Omega Point.

Additional Fresh Wisdom Axioms

In Chapter 12, The Fresh Wisdom Ethos, we introduced 12 Axioms by which all *Fresh Thinkers* lead their life. Instead of repeating all 12 Axioms, here are two which are relevant to this discussion:

Axiom #8 – Purpose

The uninitiated masses almost never know their real reasons for doing anything. *Fresh Thinkers*, in contrast, never accept anything without questioning and understanding it. They also understand that their life has a purpose, even though their purpose may not yet have been fully defined or understood.

Axiom #9 – Religion

Religions and cults are man-made inventions designed to allow an elitist priesthood to con value out of those that follow them. *Fresh Thinkers* do not blindly follow any man-made religion.

In addition to the 12 Axioms already covered, there are two additional Axioms which are required to assist in reaching the Omega Point. These are:

Axiom # 13 – Biblical World View

A *Fresh Thinker* accepts without question the Biblical World View and that the only scientifically, empirically proven source document is the Bible. This book is not at variance with any proven scientific fact and shows an internal concordance of knowledge of the world of science which the initial writers could not have had, except for its inspiration by an Outside Mind. The Biblical World View is thus the only scientifically proven paradigm (way of looking at life), and thus represents a stable pyramid.

Axiom # 14 – Modern Science Distorts the Biblical Message

A *Fresh Thinker* understands that the theme of the Bible is that of a gigantic Cosmic conflict between positive and negative forces. We therefore accept that any distortion of the Biblical World View is accomplished by negative forces intent on preventing the achievement of a personal Omega Point.

These are powerful axioms, and no doubt come as a surprise considering the material we have already covered on religions. But remember, we were discussing man-made religions, not the Bible. We include Christianity in the stable of man-made religions, even though we are acknowledging the Bible as the only reliable source document.

Sounds contradictory, does not it? Let us look a little deeper. We are going to have to skim over certain profound principles in the next few pages, in the interests of keeping this chapter concise. However, we make far more detailed scientific evidence available in our publication: *The Greater Picture: Truth, Freedom and Omega Point.*[142]

Biblical World View Compared to Major Religions

We must ask, yet again, for you to put aside any pre-conditioning you may have about any religion. Remember that whatever religion you may have followed to date (including not following any religion) is a con. This will be challenging, since we are asking you to consider the Bible as a science handbook, instead of a religious text. If you have followed no particular religion to date, you may have difficulty accepting the use of the Bible as the source document. If you have 'been religious' to date, you may find some of the concepts we are about to cover difficult to accept, because you have never heard them before. If at any time your comfort zone feels threatened, go back and read The Triangular Theory of Consciousness on page 189.

Remember, what we are trying to achieve is your personal Omega Point, and no religion to date has facilitated that process.

~~~

Side Note: At the risk of repeating ourselves, the following discussion has nothing to do with Christianity, or any other religion. It has everything to do with Science, Quantum Physics, the E5 and the Omega Point. The only way you can benefit from the discussion is to remove any religious preconceptions (pre-conditioning) that will cloud your understanding.

~~~

If we were to summarize the one key difference between the world's major religions[143], it would be thus:

Jesus Christ is the only being to have materialized from another dimension into this dimension, and then returned to the dimension He came from.

While there are significant similarities between major religions, this one fact is what sets the Biblical World View apart from any other belief system. The impact of this feat has a direct bearing on achieving your personal Omega Point. Let us examine why, using science as our base.

Quantum Physics

In plain English, Quantum Physics (also called Quantum Mechanics) is the study of the really, really small sub-particles that make up atoms.

---

[142] www.freedomtechnology.org/resources/truth/omega.htm
[143] www.everystudent.com/features/connecting.html

School physics teach that the three smallest particles of matter are the proton, neutron and electron. Today, Quantum Physicists have discovered a multitude of yet smaller particles that make up atoms, called quarks, leptons, gluons, neutrinos, muons and other even stranger sounding names.

But the strangest, inexplicable thing about these tiny particles is the manner in which they behave, since these particles do not obey all previously known scientific laws – they operate randomly, and scientists do not like randomness.

At times they behave like particles (by vibrating) and at times like waves (by oscillating).

These particles often disappear, and no-one has been able to identify where they disappear to – some say they disappear into a parallel Universe.

These particles have also been shown to appear in two or more places simultaneously.

In short, scientists are somewhat baffled, and no-one has yet been able to provide a succinct explanation for Quantum Physics, or how it affects our daily lives. But many have understood that there is a powerful secret hidden in Quantum Physics. Niels Bohr has said "Those who are not shocked when they first come across quantum mechanics cannot possibly have understood it."[144]

Some have stated that Quantum Physics is a physics of possibilities, meaning that reality could exist in different forms at the same time. Others have gone further to say that Quantum Physics proves the existence of parallel realities and that these particles alternate between different forms of reality.

Others have gone as far as demonstrating by neuroscience and psychophysics that we do not perceive the world as it actually is, but as the brain computes it most probably to be. In other words, two people surveying the same environment perceive things differently. Which one is experiencing 'reality'?

"I think it is safe to say that no one understands quantum mechanics." - Richard Feynman.[145]

Needless to say, this is a confusing study of science, given our current understanding. Want to try it for yourself? Here's a good place to start: *A Lazy Layman's Guide to Quantum Physics.* [146]

The Bible and Quantum Physics

In Chapter 12 we went to some lengths to explain the scientific basis of the Bible. Many have tried to scientifically *disprove* the Bible, and yet

[144] www.spaceandmotion.com/quantum-physics-niels-bohr-quotes.htm
[145] www.banned-books.com/truth-seeker/1995archive/122_3/20realityquantum.html
[146] http://higgo.com/quantum/laymans.htm

it has stood the test of time by <u>not once</u> being at variance with any proven scientific fact.

We also concluded that the individual authors credited with writing separate books in the Bible could not have written what they did without Divine Guidance. It would then be a natural conclusion that the Bible is ultimately authored by the same Creator who brought this Universe into existence. It would stand to reason, then, that the same author wrote the rules for Quantum Physics, and already understands what scientists are grappling with right now. The author understands the concept of 'parallel realities', since this is part of the Creator's creation.

We are going to repeat that last thought, because it is important to comprehend before going further (you are going to be shocked in the next section).

The Creator wrote the rules for Quantum Physics, and already understands what scientists are grappling with right now. The Creator understands the concept of 'parallel realities', since this is part of the Creator's Universe.

Jesus and Quantum Physics

In Chapter 12 we touched on Jesus' Secret Message by providing an article written by someone who has nothing to do with Freedom Technology. We introduced the concept to prepare your mind for the fact that perhaps Jesus came to earth for a reason very different for that taught by Christianity. The theory of a bicameral mind, which was used as the basis for the article, is far from proven or accepted by a wide range of specialists in the field of mind and brain development. This theory is sometimes a useful tool to demonstrate some aspects, but not a conclusive or proven theory.

But back to our point, it does appear as if the person of Jesus was carrying a secret message. What could that secret be?

Here is a profound thought – profound because it relates directly to our reaching the Omega Point.

Jesus Christ came to this earth to prove Quantum Physics. He did this by materializing from another dimension (a parallel Universe?) into this dimension. He showed us that there is another version of reality (by walking on water, by raising the dead, by turning water into wine and by performing other miracles which contradict the known scientific laws in *this* dimension).

Quantum Physicists agree that, theoretically and based on the behavior of sub-atomic particles, it should be possible to walk on water. And this is precisely what Jesus proved more than 2,000 years ago! He came with a secret message: to prove that another dimension does exist – the same concept Quantum Physicists are struggling with right now.

Jesus did not come to 'save mankind from their sins', as we have been taught to believe by man-made religions, but to prove that we can create our own reality – again, this is a concept Quantum Physicists are grappling with right now

This is getting a little heavy, so let us back up a little.

Freedom Technology and Quantum Physics

There are a few core *Fresh Wisdom* Axioms which bear repeating at this point. This is to encourage you to think for yourself, instead of simply accepting another man-made 'religion'.

Axiom #1 – Reducing Controls

In order to become free, a *Fresh Thinker* greatly reduces the external controls placed on their life. They will not allow themselves to be controlled by anyone (including Freedom Technology).

Understand that we are not forcing any controlling thought process on you. Rather, we are encouraging you to think about the existence of a reality which is different to what has already been forced on you.

Axiom #2 – Avoid Con Artists

Con artists seek to maximize the volume of life's pleasures which flow their way, by conning money, energy, time and talent from other people.

What we have just stated (that Jesus came not to save mankind from their sins, but to prove Quantum Physics) may not be true, but we believe it implicitly after years of careful study. We encourage you to critically examine this claim, as we absolutely do not wish to impose another con on you. We encourage you to listen for the ring of truth, and test everything you have read to date.

Axiom #6 – Rules and Regulations

Fresh Thinkers live by their own set of rational, coherent and internally generated rules, which may, or may not agree with the externally imposed laws.

We are not in any way forcing you to accept any new paradigms or rules. What you choose to do with this information is entirely up to you and your conscience.

Axiom #9 – Religion

Religions and cults are man-made inventions designed to allow an elitist priesthood to con value out of those that follow them. *Fresh Thinkers* do not blindly follow any man-made religion.

Please understand that we are not in the process of introducing a new religion for which we are seeking followers from whom we can con value. We are however interested in opening eyes and stimulating independent thought. The field of Quantum Physics is a profoundly exciting study, made many times more so when Jesus' life and miracles are introduced into the equation.

Axiom #11 – Responsibility

Responsibility for what happens in the life of a *Fresh Thinker* rests solely with that individual.

Responsibility now does lie with you as to what your reaction will be. You can either reject these thoughts outright, or choose to investigate for yourself whether there may be some validity in them. Whatever your choice, there will be consequences.

In short, we have reminded you of these axioms so that you are 100% convinced that we are not trying to force a con on you.

The Matrix

You may be familiar with the 1999 movie, *The Matrix*,[147] starring Keanu Reeves as Neo and Laurence Fishburne as Morpheus. This is by far the best fictional explanation of the concept we are trying to explain. If you have not seen the movie, we highly encourage you to do so, as it will help come to grips with the concept of a parallel Universe and Quantum Physics. (Sequels to *The Matrix I* seem to have lost the plot with regards to Quantum Physics – perhaps the writers were forced to drop their otherwise profound message.)

Very briefly, the movie is about a computer hacker who learns from mysterious rebels about the true nature of his reality and his role in the war against the controllers of it. But the underlying plot and storyline are far more profound. You may previously have read articles on religious messages embedded in *The Matrix*, but these[148] are nothing compared to what you are about to read now. Do not worry, we will not give the plot away – we will simply quote from the movie.

Quotes from The Matrix

NEO: "I know what you are trying to do!"

MORPHEUS: "I am trying to free your mind, Neo. But I can only show you the door. You are the one that has to walk through it. You have to let it all go, Neo: fear, doubt and disbelief. Free your mind!"

~~~

Is that not what Jesus came to do – free us from the bondage of the law? Free us from artificial systems that enslave us? Free us from those who wish to control us? And even Jesus only ever showed his audience the door. The choice was always left to the individual as to what action to take. Allowing freedom of choice is the greatest expression of love any individual can show.

---

[147] www.imdb.com/title/tt0133093/

[148] http://atheism.about.com/library/FAQs/religion/blrel_matrix.htm

NEO: "This isn't real?"

MORPHEUS: "What is real? How do you define real? If you are talking about your senses, what you feel, taste, smell, or see; then all you are talking about are electrical signals interpreted by your brain."

More and more, Quantum Physicists are beginning to accept that reality is purely what the observer's brain chooses to interpret. They tell us that the average brain processes 400 billion pieces of information per second, but we are only aware of 2,000. Where is the other reality represented by the remaining 399 billion and some pieces of information? Perhaps in a parallel Universe – an alternate reality?

MORPHEUS: "You are here because you know something. What you know, you cannot explain. You felt it your entire life. There is something wrong with the world. You do not know what it is, but it is there, like a splinter in your mind, driving you mad. It is this feeling that has brought you to me. Do you know what I am talking about?"

NEO: "The Matrix?"

MORPHEUS: "Do you want to know what it is? Have you ever had a dream, that you were so sure was real? What if you were unable to wake from that dream? How would you know the difference between the Dream world and the Real world?"

By now you are aware of the con of the world we live in. Imagine if we could wake up from this dream, and step into the real world? Reverse roles just for a moment. Remember the last vivid (enjoyable) dream you had? What if THAT was the real world, and this is the dream world? This is not science fiction – highly intelligent professors, academics, philosophers and scientists are spending billons of dollars to get to the bottom of this. If they are taking this so seriously, shouldn't you?

MORPHEUS: "The Matrix is everywhere, it is all around us, here even in this room. You can see it out of your window, or on your television. You feel it when you go to work, or go to church, or pay your taxes. It is the world that has been pulled over your eyes to blind you from the truth."

NEO: "What truth?"

MORPHEUS: "That you are a slave, Neo. That you, like everyone else, was born into bondage. . . kept inside a prison that you cannot smell, or touch. A prison for your mind. Unfortunately no one can be told what the Matrix is. You have to see it for yourself."

~~~

Has *Fresh Wisdom* helped you see the real-world matrix for yourself? We are now going far beyond identifying the cons we have already covered. Can you see that, even though you have become significantly more enlightened than when you began, you are STILL trapped in only one Universe, when there exist many parallel Universes? Mmmm, this is becoming stranger and stranger.

~~~

MORPHEUS: "What is the Matrix? Control. The Matrix is a computer generated Dreamworld built to keep us under control, in order to change a human being into a battery of energy. We are the energy source easily renewable and completely recyclable. All they needed to control this mind was something to occupy our mind. And they built a prison out of our past; wired it to our brain and turned us into slaves."

~~~

Forget for a moment the sci-fi setting of the movie, and apply this to your life. Have you not been controlled by all manner of distractions? And we are not talking about the obvious distractions like TV and sport. What about your religion? Your hobbies? Your friends? Your political involvement? Your salaried position? Any activity which occupies your mind is potentially a distraction placed there to control your mind.

~~~

MORPHEUS: "The Matrix is a system, Neo. That system is our enemy. When you are inside you look around. What do you see? Teachers, lawyers, businessmen: the very minds of the people that we are trying to save. But until we do, these people are still a part of that system. You have to understand most of these people are not ready to be unplugged and many of them are so inert, so hopelessly dependent on the system, that they will fight any change."

~~~

Remember Axiom 4 – All Are Not Equal? Be careful who you share this information with, unless you are prepared for your audience to 'fight any change'.

~~~

HEAD AGENT ['the baddie' - pointing to our modern society]: "Have you ever stared at it? Marvel at its beauty, its genius? Billions of people living their lives - oblivious. Do you know that the first Matrix was designed to be a perfect human world, with no suffering, where everyone would be happy? It was a disaster. No one would accept the program. Entire crops were lost. Some believed that we lacked the programming language to define the perfect world."

HEAD AGENT: Do you hear Morpheus? I am going to be honest with you. I hate this place. This zoo. This prison. This reality. I must get out of here. I must get free.

~~~

Is getting free of this reality not what you must do? Could it be that Jesus came to show us just how to do so and that there is another reality to escape to?

~~~

NEO: What are you trying to tell me, that I can dodge bullets?
MORPHEUS: No Neo. I'm trying to tell you that when you are ready, you will not have to.

~~~

That is the mindset that *Fresh Wisdom* is encouraging you to adopt. Not to fight the system, not to dodge the tax man, not to resist the New World Order[149] or any other form of globalization. Simply play life by your own rules. Avoid situations where bullets may be flying around in slow motion, not dodge them.

There are many more quotes we could use from the movie, but you probably get the point. We have intentionally left out two or three particularly juicy quotes that will send shivers down your spine when you watch the movie with this mindset. Even if you have seen it a dozen times before, go and watch this movie as soon as you can!

Why is Jesus' Message a Secret?

At this point a number of obvious questions raise their ugly heads:
- Why have religions not made the connection between Jesus, the science of the Bible, Quantum Physics, parallel realities and the Omega Point?
- What is the short-cut to the Omega Point?
- Why is the message secret, or why is it made so difficult for us to understand?

There are three reasons for this.

Reason 1 – Conflict Between Positive and Negative

Does it not make sense that in the Cosmic battle between Positive and Negative, Good and Evil, Yin and Yang, that the negative force will employ every means possible to keep us from reaching the point of ultimate understanding? The battle that is in progress has as its focus, control of our minds.

If the positive force were to step in and right these wrongs, would that not be removing the element of free choice – the freedom of choice being the greatest display of love?

Reason 2 – Proving Responsibility

---

[149] www.threeworldwars.com/nwo.htm

Handing the keys to understanding of the power of Jesus' message to any unqualified individual is akin to handing the keys to your brand new motor vehicle to a 16-year old teenage boy, together with a bottle of vodka and an invitation to 'have fun'.

We are to prove our responsibility, and our commitment to do something with the information, before full understanding is given to us.

Accordingly, a giant obstacle course has been laid out before us, including the entire collection of con's we have been subject to. Our ability to step out of our comfort zone and navigate through the obstacle course is what proves our commitment.

Reason 3 – The Process of Preparation

There is no short-cut to the Omega Point. Do not for a minute think that by reading to the end of this chapter you will have reached your personal Omega Point. The journey and the lessons learnt along the way are far more important than the destination. The reason we are currently in this dimension is for training in preparation for the next dimension. Training in understanding and control of the Universe and dealing with the two forces of positive and negative that are inherent in the system.

What we have tried to do is provide a map to speed the process of finding the start of the Omega Point. The rest of the journey is totally up to you, although we will help as far as this is possible.

Reaching the Omega Point

The Omega Point. Does it exist? Is it attainable? If so, where and when?

Jesus said to him, I am the Way and the Truth and the Life.[150]

So, it appears that absolute Truth does exist somewhere. But can we attain to it?

And you will know the Truth, and the Truth will set you free.[151]

Therefore let us go on and get past the elementary stage in the teachings and doctrine of Christ (the Messiah), advancing steadily toward the completeness and perfection that belong to spiritual maturity.[152]

His intention was the perfecting and the full equipping of the saints (His consecrated people), [that they should do] the work of ministering toward building up Christ's body (the church), [That it might develop] until we all attain oneness in the faith and in the comprehension of the [full and accurate] knowledge of the Son of God, that [we might arrive] at really mature

---

[150] John 14:6
[151] John 8:32
[152] Hebrews 6:1

manhood (the completeness of personality which is nothing less than the standard height of Christ's own perfection), the measure of the stature of the fullness of the Christ and the completeness found in Him.[153]

It appears that we can attain the truth.

When Will We Reach The Omega Point?

And I am convinced and sure of this very thing, that He Who began a good work in you will continue until the day of Jesus Christ [right up to the time of His return], developing [that good work] and perfecting and bringing it to full completion in you[154].

It is a process. Some attain to different levels. We are all at our personal positions along the way. But it appears that it may not be attained in this lifetime. Solomon was one individual who progressed very far on this journey.

How Do We Reach The Omega Point?

This is why I was born, and for this I have come into the world, to bear witness to the Truth. Everyone who is of the Truth [who is a friend of the Truth, who belongs to the Truth] hears and listens to My voice.[155]

But when He, the Spirit of Truth (the Truth-giving Spirit) comes, He will guide you into all the Truth (the whole, full Truth).[156]

If any of you is deficient in wisdom, let him ask of the giving God [Who gives] to everyone liberally and ungrudgingly, without reproaching or faultfinding, and it will be given him.[157]

So, it appears, unless He specifically chooses you to be able to understand Truth, tough luck! You may, of course, ask. (And that would be acknowledging He exists.)

This may seem totally unreasonable, but remember Axiom 7 – Fairness? A *Fresh Thinker* understands and accepts that the world is and always will be an unfair place. We do not squander energy debating why this is – we simply accept it as a given.

Why Aim for The Omega Point?

The beginning of Wisdom is: get Wisdom! [For skilful and godly Wisdom is the principal thing.][158]

---

[153] Ephesians 4:12-13
[154] Philippians 1:6
[155] John 18:37
[156] John 16:13
[157] James 1:5

The reverent and worshipful fear of the Lord [actually believing in Him] is the beginning (the chief and choice part) of Wisdom, and the knowledge of the Holy One is insight and understanding.[159]

But rather what we are setting forth is a wisdom of God once hidden [from the human understanding] and now revealed to us by God--[that wisdom] which God devised and decreed before the ages for our glorification [to lift us into the glory of His presence].[160]

If the Truth will set us free, what is freedom?

The Meaning of Freedom

The freedom Jesus offers is far more than the freedom achieved through political or revolutionary methods. It is freedom from the state of bondage to sin (the matrix) in which all human beings find themselves,[161] freedom from domination by the fallen angel Satan,[162] and freedom from every aspect of death.[163] That is the kind of freedom which is offered by Christ - which lasts not only in this life but for all eternity. This is a truly revolutionary freedom - infinitely transcending anything which governments or guerrilla leaders can offer.

It presents a purpose to this life: preparation for a future existence in an expanded dimension.

Where Do We Find This Freedom?

Your Word is Truth.[164]

It appears we can start with His Word. Then the Force takes over at some point. So, we must start with the Bible.

As the proofs of past foretelling of events and their fulfillment have been evidence of His control, so future events will be demonstrated to tie in with the predicted in such a way as to leave absolutely no doubt of the inter-connectedness within, and the reality of, the Quantum Spectrum and its absolutes of pre-planning and ordering of the Universe, by an Outside-of-the-System Initiator.

Get to know Him better through His unique Message (the Bible) to *you*, His Greatest Miracle! Discover your real self. Welcome to Ultimate Reality. You have been presented with the Omega Point. Now what are you going to do with it?

---

[158] Proverbs 4:7
[159] Proverbs 9:10
[160] 1 Corinthians 2:7
[161] John 8:34-36, 41-44
[162] 1 John 3:8; Mark 3:27
[163] Hebrews 2:14-15
[164] John 17:17

I came that they may have and enjoy life, and have it in abundance (to the full, till it overflows).[165]

The 5 Fresh Wisdom Pillars and the Omega Point

Hopefully now it is becoming clear how every one of the 5 *Fresh Wisdom* Pillars of Fulfilled Living is essential to reaching your personal Omega Point. Each pillar is a tightly knit element in the pyramid leading to full understanding, and each Pillar interacts with others. Each Pillar must be understood fully in order to build a solid world view.

In the next few weeks, the full impact of what we have discussed thus far will become more meaningful to you, as your mind 'integrates' the various nodes we have presented. Until then, here is a reminder of the 5 Pillars, and specifically how they relate to reaching your personal Omega Point:

1. **Health & Longevity**: Once you are excited about this concept of parallel realities, you may realize that living free from pain and discomfort to at least age 120 is the very least you will want to achieve. There is so much to learn, and so little time. In addition, we may have squandered so much of our life already on frivolous activities, so there is a catch up process required. In addition, we have to prove our worth for the next Dimension, and that may take some doing – we need all the time we can get!

2. **Love-life or Relationship** principles and skills: We have already covered the significance of making love as a preparation for The Grand Affair – our love affair with God. Your relationship in this dimension has little to do with how happy you are, or how happy your partner is – it has everything to do with preparing you for the ultimate relationship when Jesus returns.

3. **Financial Freedom**: Very few employers will want to employ someone older than 65, never mind 100 or 120. So developing the skills required for a passive income is vital. In addition, your retirement fund is unlikely to continue funding your extended life sufficiently.

4. **Metaphysical Truths**: As we have hopefully shown, many metaphysical truths have been hidden from us, either by design, or because we were too lazy to go looking. Hopefully *Fresh Wisdom* has given you a new framework, a new way of looking at the world around us. Now it is your task to research further, and in so doing expand your understanding.

---

[165] John 10:10

5. **Sovereignty and Privacy** strategies: Hopefully we have shown just how fickle man-made laws are. But we are still required to live in this repressive society and obey the laws of the land. The mindset you have now achieved is one that will allow you to remain relatively unseen – under the radar – as you go about your new life purpose.

As you can see, the 5 Pillars really are all interrelated, culminating in reaching your Personal Omega Point.

This chapter has included our most powerful principles to date, and in essence the whole point of *Fresh Wisdom*. We would be surprised if you are able to fully grasp all the concepts in one sitting – it has taken us a combined 80-person years to do so. May we suggest that you put the material aside for a few days and read it again and again. We hope that as you open your mind to this new concept you will understand what a wonderful life lies ahead of you.

~~~

No nation ancient or modern ever lost the liberty of freely speaking, writing, or publishing their sentiments, but forthwith lost their liberty in general and became slaves. – John P. Zenger

There is a wonderful mythical law of nature that the three things we crave most in life -- happiness, freedom, and peace of mind -- are always attained by giving them to someone else. - Peyton Conway March

Liberty, taking the word in its concrete sense, consists in the ability to choose. – Simone Weil

Eternal vigilance is the price of liberty. – Wendell Phillips

If you were all alone in the universe with no one to talk to, no one with which to share the beauty of the stars, to laugh with, to touch, what would be your purpose in life? It is other life, it is love, which gives your life meaning. This is harmony. We must discover the joy of each other, the joy of challenge, the joy of growth. – Mitsugi Saotome

The secret of joy in work is contained in one word - excellence. To know how to do something well is to enjoy it. – Pear l S. Buck

18. The Ten Second Miracle

The Ten Second Miracle is a logical next step from our discussion on the Omega Point.

The following article is adapted from Neo-Tech Principles[166] by Ron Robinson[167], and is a necessary exercise to complete before forging ahead to create your new wealth. While the miracle can be performed in ten seconds, it requires a fair amount of preparation, hence the preceding material in this manual.

The Ten Second Miracle

Start your journey into the eternal sunshine of a spotlessly-honest mind. In just ten seconds:
- You are going to shrink bogus authorities to vanishing points;
- You are going to shrink ignorance and superstition, orthodoxy and fundamentalism, hatred and intolerance to vanishing points;
- You are going to shrink the sociopathic duet of religion and politics to vanishing points, leaving bogus clergy, career politicians, lawyers and judges with no honor, glory, or dignity;
- You are going to eliminate dishonesty, irrationality, and injustice;
- You are going to send bogus external authorities who spiritually impoverish and then physically kill everyone to the dustbin of history;
- You are going to experience open-ended prosperity, health well into your second century, and romantic happiness;
- You are going to integrate honesty with facts in reality and natural law to undermine, and then exploit the hoax of the anti-civilization destruction, and discover personal powers to build a civilization of open ended prosperity and happiness;
- You are going to change your views, and your psychology. Your new powers of consciousness are going to come from linear-digital processing, not from the circular-analog thinking of a reality that was created for you
- You are going break free of and eliminate parasitical external authority induced mysticisms that undermine both your short and long range prospects for joy and happiness. This external authority is achieved through a bizarrely irrational transfer of your value production to a handful of elite for obscene unearned power, glory, and wealth. This wealth is obtained not by producing values, but by usurping and draining billions via a fictional mind-created false economy designed to rob you of the wealth derived from your

[166] www.neo-tech.com/
[167] http://americanfreeenterprise.blogspot.com/

productive efforts, while ravaging entire industries, businesses, and professions;

- By removing excess body weight you are going to free up energy you did not realize you had, and easily accomplish tasks that previously seemed difficult because of the unnecessary expenditures of energy spent maneuvering over mountains of mind created realities, by shrinking them into trivial nonsense points with no basis in reality;
- You are going to start growing more youthful;
- You are going to remove unnecessary and contrived guilt foisted upon your shoulders by malevolent criminal-minded individuals whose survival depends on coercive manipulations of truths by usurping your natural thinking process and productive efforts for their malevolent unearned power, unreal wealth, and unearned glory. They will vanish into the dustbin;
- You are going to dump mystical altruisms that rob you of your natural power and return to that incorruptible child of the past to discover the life you were meant to live, and discover a new vehicle for ultimate longevity, unlimited liberty, and happiness;
- You are going to experience an increase in your productive capabilities by eliminating unnatural reliance on external mystical beliefs propagated by incestuously corrupt and religious, political, and educational institutions, and will gain power to accomplish difficult tasks easily as your power of free agency self-determinism is released by breaking down non-existent mind created barriers that turn you into fearful conformists and prevent you from achieving your potential by stifling your ability to create limitless wealth and happiness through mystic-free value production and wealth creation;
- You are going to gain the power to identify facts in reality, easily recognize previously conceived obstacles not as barriers, but valuable assets to be exploited to find solutions that provide ever-increasing values for mankind, and that allow you to easily move around these mind-created obstacles to solve problems while others struggle in their attempts to overcome the obstructions that have been created for them, and prevent their forward progress, and then out-compete others in all areas of life.

But first, we need to identify the anti-civilization matrix that holds you back from a guiltless pursuit of life, liberty, and happiness. To fix the vehicle, it is first necessary to identify the faulty components that bring the vehicle to a halt. Below are some of those faulty components of the anti-civilization matrix:

Educational Systems in which tax exempt foundations rewrite history according to the latest liar or victor and teach children to integrate into a disintegrating society designed to reduce civilization to the lowest common denominator in a master-slave relationship on a global plantation, and force-funded by usurpations of earned wealth and property rights through forced legal tenant/rent type taxation schemes and bogus force-backed laws that demand subservience against the will of the individual majority backed by the illegitimate use of force by uncontrolled political and legal institutions backed by subjective law and forced at the end of a barrel by duped individuals in law enforcement in a democracy where 51 percent of the population is allowed to tell 49 percent of the population what to do, and how to run their lives, and the lives of their children. Some of the most successful and productive members of society never completed government-forced educational systems, thus freeing them to create extraordinary values for themselves, and society.

Religious Systems that render eternal progression hostage to a violent god or allah and by foisting guilt on innocent victims through manipulated 'truths' by individuals seeking unearned power and control at the expense of the righteous and unalienable pursuit of life, liberty, and happiness in a bizarrely unnatural anti-civilization in the pursuit of a questionable afterlife virtually unobtainable by disobedience of the immutable laws of the Universe, and which ultimately culminates in the loss of life of all the inhabitants of planet Earth if allowed to continue on its present course.

Energy Systems designed to hold us hostages to Oil Company profiteers with no hope for free energy or renewable energy abundantly available throughout existence, but denied by malevolent greed at the expense of your unalienable natural rights.

Income Taxation and Property Taxation that transfers individual power and wealth creation to a malevolent handful of elite who use bogus monetary systems created out of nothing of any tangible value, and used to gain unlimited control of the masses to accomplish their malevolent agenda of a feudalistic master-slave relationship on a global plantation in a mathematically formulated model consisting of only those individual servants necessary to maintain their utopian goals of no-effort wealth, power, and dominion at the expense of the natural law rights of every conscious individual on the planet.

Our false buying power fueled by the endless creation of debt using paper money systems few are able to comprehend, unwittingly held hostage to cheap products from hostage labor in foreign countries made possible only by the exportation of debt by forced political subservience from the hostage countries manipulated by illegitimate governments and controlled career politicians who unwittingly transfer power to elite and corporate interests, for the purpose of gain derived from a house of cards designed to self-destruct to accomplish the dual purpose of war profiteering and population reduction strategies.

The Emerging Global Police State resulting from increasingly tyrannical governments now holding us hostage by, among others, Patriot Act 1 and 2; through usurpation of our voting power in a constitutional republic usurped by transforming political institutions into a one party system of hypocrisy which serves only the rich and corporate interests by transforming prosperity enhancing republican forms of government into no-win democratic systems that factual history demonstrate perennially fall when individuals discover they can vote themselves largess from the public funds, and as history shows, ultimately devolve into communist socialist fascist government systems at the expense of the many for the benefit of the few by manipulating facts in reality in ways that the majority, driven by misguided pride and the pursuit of no-effort unearned wealth are unaware that such a system is inimical to their best interests until the system collapses under its own weight and the people are left without resources to control their destiny.

A Bogus War on Terrorism propagated by terrorist regimes using inversions of reality whereby duped masses operating in an upside down anti-civilization psychologically conditioned to cognize evil as good, and good as evil.

And where did they get all this power to control our lives?

WE GAVE IT TO THEM!

Are you ready to take back control? Control of your mind?

Are you ready to cure the disease that created problems where none exist, and lethally blights human consciousness?

Are you ready to start your journey into the eternal sunshine of a spotlessly-honest mind?

Do you have ten seconds?

Before we give you the key, we need to give you a few instructions about how this vehicle operates. It is going to take a little effort, or discipline on your part; which usually always involves doing something you least want to do - like *work*, or *facing reality*. You might have to skip a meal or two. You might have to skip your favorite television program, the controlled media news, or heaven forbid; your favorite sporting event. You might even consider skipping church. You are going to have to get out of your comfort zone, and you can accomplish in just ten seconds what has taken others years of research and thought to learn and comprehend.

You are going to have to learn to use your brain all over again. You are going take back your mind by allowing it to integrate *facts* in *reality*. You are going to have to *think*.

The miracle will not happen unless *you make it happen.* You are going to have to take *action.* You cannot create something by doing nothing. But what will probably be the hardest obstacle you will encounter as you begin to operate the vehicle, is that you are going to have to be completely *honest* with yourself in all areas of life.

You are going to have to learn to accept responsibility for your actions. You are going to have to realize that the use of force, fraud, and coercion are never justified, and realize that real wealth comes not as a gift, but from hard, disciplined effort in accordance with natural law, because in ten seconds you are about to harness power you never knew you had, and with power comes responsibility.

Are you ready? You are about to escape this reality and explode out the other side into a civilization 180 degrees parallel to one you are now in. At the end of the journey you will find yourself outside the anti-civilization bubble looking in. You are going to see things as you have never seen them before.

Are you ready?

We are going to use the following quote by Robert Thayer to describe the process:

"If the number of errors in a number of lines of code is a known quantity, an Engineer would not try to repair or improve some poorly designed software by adding more lines of code. Subtractive thinking must be employed: make a system work by taking something away. In the case of software this would directly reduce the number of errors."

OK. Do you have ten seconds?

We are going to hand over the key that opens the door. You are about to enter the vehicle that is going to take you places you have yet to imagine. You are about to remove the 'faulty lines of code'.

First, take a few minutes to form a mental picture of practically everything you have ever been taught from your earliest memory to the present moment. Imagine your whole life flashing before you in a high speed motion picture film, and freeze it into a single frame.

Take a deep breath, deep into your lungs, hold it for a brief moment, and let it out with a sigh.

Do this three times.

Now take the picture you are holding in your mind, and DUMP IT. Hit the button, and send it to the recycle bin! Do not worry about it - you can always retrieve it from the recycle bin, although we do not know why anyone would want to do that. Trust us, the anti-civilization will still be there trying to suck you back in.

Ten seconds, every time.

Welcome to the civilization of the Universe. Enjoy the ride!

19. True Value Creation

We have mentioned 'true value creation' a few times in preceding pages, and the reason we introduced *The Ten Second Miracle* at this point is because we would like you to forget any wealth creation strategies you may have come across before that 'contain lines of faulty code'. Let us be honest, wealth creation plays right into the hands of those wanting to extract value from those driven by greed. You can see this in the way classified ads, magazine advertorials and seminars for Wealth Creation or Wealth Management courses are advertised. We have all heard the phrase 'Get Rich Quick' so often that it is now only used together with the word 'scheme'. There is no such thing as 'Get Rich Quick', which is why we are asking you to dump any preconceived ideas you may have about 'instant' wealth creation.

What we are talking about now is a wealth creation method which supports all the *Fresh Wisdom* Axioms and Principles. We wanted to create an opportunity which is 100% ethical because it focuses on true value creation instead of conning values from an unsuspecting, gullible market. Let us remind ourselves what the laws are.

The Laws of Financial Independence & Wealth Creation are based on:

Materialization: This is a fundamental law of the Universe: what the mind of man can conceive, it can bring about. The mind is the workshop in which everything is initially created.

Persistence: Without persistence, very little is ever achieved. With it, anything can be accomplished. Understanding and harnessing it can lead to the achievement of any goal. A Plan without Persistence is no plan at all.

Actualization: The ultimate reason and purpose for a successful life is to attain transcendent self-actualization. This is what we refer to as the Omega Point. Self-actualization is to find self-fulfillment and realize one's full potential. Self-transcendence is to connect to something beyond the ego or to help others find self-fulfillment and realize their potential.

Leverage: This law is the principle of taking all of your assets (your time being the most valuable) and making them work for you.

Let us discuss each in a little more detail.

Materialization

The concept behind *Fresh Wisdom* is to stimulate creative, independent thought. As you progressed through the manual you no doubt thought of better ways of explaining some of the concepts. Many even think of totally new concepts, triggered by something explained in *Fresh Wisdom*.

Over the next few weeks more and more concepts will crystallize in your mind, and it is not uncommon for people to wake in the middle of the night with yet another "Aha!" experience as something clicks into place.

We suggest you keep a record of these 'revelations'. Each revelation on their own may not mean too much to you right now, but after a series of such 'mind parties' something wonderful starts to happen: a concrete idea for how you can help others materializes from the dim mists. This idea will form the first product which will start building your Independent Wealth Creation System. More about this a little later.

Freedom Technology materialized in just this manner. Three people got together with the vaguest of ideas, and absolutely no idea how to make it work. All we could ever come up with were the obstacles and challenges in making this information available to a wide audience. But there is power in 'sending a message into the Universe'. Perhaps it has to do with those parallel realities we discussed earlier. Perhaps the Creator does respond to such requests (note that we are not referring to the pious forms of prayer many religions teach). Whatever the reason, the fact that you are reading this information proves that the Law of Materialization is real and it works.

Persistence

Persistence is defined as 'to try to do or continue doing something in a determined but often unreasonable way'.

Needless to say, there is a difference between persisting with a plan doomed to failure and following a dream which is grounded in Natural Law. *Fresh Wisdom* has shown you what the basis is of Natural Law, and any product ideas grounded in these laws have traditionally achieved success in the past, given the required persistence and dedication.

A perfect example of dedicated persistence is Einstein, who is said to have conducted more than 9,000 experiments to perfect the light bulb. See *4 Lessons in Creativity* online.[168]

The difference with persistence when applied to the Freedom Technology Wealth Creation Model, is that the results achieved are long term. This is completely different to 'persisting' in a salaried position where your only reward is a token salary payment at the end of the month.

---

[168] www.newsscan.com/exec/spring1998/4lessons.html

Actualization

Here is a statement that may sound harsh: 'Unless you reach your Personal Omega Point, any product you create will be conning value from the market.'

Look, it is easy to make money these days on the Internet. We can quote many examples of unscrupulous marketers who take information already in the public domain, package it into an eBook, craft a slick sales letter (or they pay someone else to do it for them) and make money – often truckloads of it. That is not value creation – it is value extraction.

The reason people do this is because without reaching the Omega Point, there really is nothing new under the sun. The sheeple are so caught in the bubble of their anti-civilization that creative thought is impossible. So they resort to repackaging the same information. And the sheeple fall for it, because they know no better.

However, after reaching your Omega Point, *new* ideas are generated and triggered, and it is these ideas which create value, and which will form the basis of any products in your Wealth Creation System.

Leverage

As we have said before, the best known example of leverage is that of pop stars or authors, who apply effort once (recording an album, writing a book) and continue earning income for years after, every time an album or book is sold. Until you can leverage your time, you will never become wealthy and powerful. As we have explained in previous chapters, we will be using the Internet to continue selling a product you have created for many years after you have made the initial commitment.

But we will be leveraging an additional system, which we will explain now.

A surprising (to us) side-effect of *Fresh Wisdom* is the hunger for more information. "How can that be?" we kept lamenting. "We wanted to create the complete guide for Fulfilled Living, and yet we are receiving hundreds of questions wanting to know more!"

But that is perfectly in-line with our desire to stimulate creative thinking, and we are pleased to see how many have contacted us wanting clarification on certain concepts. And it is this hunger which creates a perfect opportunity for you. The *Fresh Wisdom* concept is still very new, and it would help us tremendously if you could expound a particular principle. In doing so, you will have started your own wealth creation system.

So, you will be leveraging the Freedom Technology Community. Would you not feel more comfortable buying information from someone you know has read this manual? That is exactly what other *Fresh Thinkers* have been telling us. In this way we can all work together to increase 'collective consciousness' of the *Fresh Wisdom* concepts.

Incidentally, this community is not a feeble gathering of a few hundred people. This manual and the Freedom Technology Email Seminar has enjoyed significant growth, and we have even bigger plans to grow significantly. Our conservative aim is 10 million free Seminars distributed by the end of 2007, the majority of whom will remain part of the community because of the ongoing value gained. So, as you can see, you will be leveraging a pretty powerful community! A community all dedicated to value creation, not value extraction.

You are obviously under no obligation whatsoever to leverage this system. There is enough information in the Wealth Creation Seminars to go off on your own, if you so wish. However, we have found that a helping hand every now and then certainly eases the learning curve, and we hope you will take advantage of this system.

How Does the FT Wealth Creation System Work?

Just a reminder: At no point will you be working for, on behalf of, or for the benefit of Freedom Technology. We are not some sort of Multi Level Marketing (MLM) organization. You will be keeping everything you make as a result of implementing these strategies.

Very simply, you write a digital downloadable eBook explaining one or more concepts of *Fresh Wisdom*, we market it for you, you keep all revenue generated by sales of your eBook. You win by building your Wealth Creation System, and we win by having the concepts of *Fresh Wisdom* expanded far quicker than this small team of three people can accomplish. The arrangement works on the principles of Axiom #12 – Relationships: Successful relationships hinge upon a continued and approximately equal exchange of values between the partners. When an imbalance occurs the imbalance is addressed or the relationship is ended.

The system itself is only due to launch in Quarter 1, 2006, as we are still developing all the supporting material required to make this truly effective. But that does not mean you cannot start writing your book right now, so that by the time we are ready, you could be one of the first to use this incredible system.

Responsibilities

Perhaps the best method of explaining who is responsible for which part of your Wealth Creation System is by means of a table.

Responsibilities for Each Party in the FT Wealth Creation System	
Fresh Thinker	Freedom Technology
Create the product, including proof-reading, final editing and conversion to pdf	Provide advice and guidance in the selection of a product idea
Write a compelling sales letter and follow up sequence (or mini-course)*	Provide a once-off Launch Announcement to the FT Community (by email)
Handle all prospect queries, customer complaints and refund requests *	Make reference to the product at appropriate places in the Email Seminar Series and other publications
Register with a payment processor to handle online payments	Include the product and brief description in the FT Shopping Cart, with a direct link to your sales letter
Provide additional marketing for external prospects (pay-per-click ads, etc. – if required)	Set up auto-responders and follow-up sequences for prospects
Register a domain name and arrange hosting *	Track performance and provide reports on a monthly basis.

* We will very soon be offering a service whereby the more technical aspects of the system can be handled by us. There will be a small charge for this service, as this is a true value creation service for someone who may not want to concern themselves with technicalities.

Frequently Asked Questions

We will soon have a detailed User Guide explaining the whole process, but until we do, here are answers to some of the questions most often asked.

1. Will FT market *anything* I produce?

You will find that we are extremely lenient regarding standards, content and even belief systems, so the short answer is Yes, we will market anything you produce (with certain exceptions obviously). However, you should be aware of a few pointers.

We strictly limit the number of Product Launch emails, to ensure that subscribers are not flooded with useless marketing messages. Priority is given to those products which: conform to and agree with the FT Philosophy; can easily be categorized into one of the 5 Pillars of Fulfilled Living; and meet certain formatting guidelines.

FT uses an Endorsement System. All products are reviewed by a panel prior to inclusion in the FT System – those that the panel agrees are in support of the FT Philosophy are assigned a special logo, indicating that it is endorsed by FT. Products that blatantly negate or challenge FT principles will be marketed with a suitable warning.

In other words, it is in your interests to prepare material largely in line with FT Principles. This is because we believe anything contradictory is value extraction, not value creation. We do reserve the right to reject material for any reason.

2. Will FT own anything I produce?

No. It is your product and everything about the product remains yours. We are simply offering to advertise your product with no further commitment on your part, and no guarantee of success on our part.

3. What type of products can be sold?

We highly recommend only producing information products. The easiest product is a digitally downloadable eBook, because this simplifies the delivery mechanism. However you may choose to produce audio cassettes or CD's, DVD's, consulting services, physical books or any other product you believe will add value and produce revenue.

4. How many pages should an eBook consist of?

Between 100 to 200 pages. The entire book should never exceed 800Kb is size, so beware of large graphics. Booklets for 20 pages are fairly common, but are usually given away as a sample for a lengthier book.

5. Who sets the price of the product?

You do, and we encourage you to change the price frequently to test the results. We recommend pricing anywhere between $17 and $97 for a digital download, depending on the value provided by the product. The price of a product can often be significantly increased by adding relevant bonuses.

Physical info products (like DVD sets and manuals) can sell for as much as $1,000, but we would recommend starting small first.

6. What payment processor should I use?

If this is the first time you are marketing on the Internet, we recommend keeping it simple (i.e. you do not need to open a Merchant Account). We recommend www.ClickBank.com or www.Paypal.com.

7. Who handles shipping and inventory for physical products?

This is entirely your responsibility, although we recommend outsourcing to a company like www.FulfillmentCentral.com.

8. Who is responsible for copyright protection and copyright infringement issues?

You are responsible for all matters relating to copyright, including any copyright infringement within your works.

9. Where can I find further answers on digital product creation?

While we would love to help you, we cannot at this stage provide further assistance on digital product creation. We encourage you to consider Michael Green's *How to Create & Sell Products Online*[169] as this will shave many weeks or months off your learning time.

General questions regarding formatting and preparing books for Publishers on Demand can be found at lulu.com[170] and booksurge.com.[171]

We hope this chapter has made you excited about starting your own Wealth Creation System. We will soon be able to provide more details, but get started on writing your book!

~~~

All religions, arts and sciences are branches of the same tree. All these aspirations are directed toward ennobling man's life, lifting it from the sphere of mere physical existence and leading the individual towards freedom. – Albert Einstein

This is the true joy in life, the being used for a purpose recognized by yourself as a mighty one; the being thoroughly worn out before you are thrown on the scrap heap; the being a force of nature instead of a feverish selfish little clod of ailments and grievances complaining that the world will not devote itself to making you happy. – George Bernard Shaw

One needs something to believe in, something for which one can have whole-hearted enthusiasm. One needs to feel that one's life has meaning, that one is needed in this world. – Hannah Senesh

Many people have a wrong idea of what constitutes true happiness. It is not attained through self-gratification, but through fidelity to a worthy purpose. – Helen Keller

---

[169] www.howtocorp.com/sales.php?offer=mbh66&pid=30
[170] www.lulu.com/help/node/view/208
[171] www.booksurgepublishing.com/info/faq.php

20. The Freedom Technology Community

We are nearing the end of this manual, but hopefully not the end of our relationship. We trust that you have enjoyed the journey as much as we have. We hope the fog has lifted and your eyes have been opened to certain fundamental delusions. We sincerely hope your life has changed in ways that could not have been described at the commencement of the journey.

This final chapter talks a little about the Freedom Technology Community and what you can expect from us in the months and years to come.

What the Future Holds for Fresh Thinkers

You will notice that this entire manual avoided any discussion of a political nature. This is because the principles covered by *Fresh Wisdom* are timeless, whereas the current political climate is fairly transient, and events develop quickly and frequently. Any comment we make today would be out of date within a week.

Throughout the manual we have presented evidence for certain facts that have been hidden from us. All throughout we have encouraged you to decide what conclusions should be drawn from each lesson. But with the current political and military climate considered, time is getting shorter for all of us. For this reason we wish to close this manual with a number of statements that may further shock you.

Self Evident Truths

During the writing of the Declaration of Independence, the authors were forced to draw some conclusions they did not have time or space to prove. They called these unsupported claims 'self evident truths,' meaning they were so obviously true that they did not need to be proved.

In a similar vein, we now offer certain blunt statements that we find to be self-evident concerning the state of the world as we write this, approaching 2006.

Self Evident Truths of the World in 2006

- We are in an era of increasing serial wars. Some have stated that World War 3 has already commenced;
- All wars have been deliberately engineered by those who profit from war, and are a physical manifestation of the spiritual battle occurring in another dimension;
- These profiteers (Warmakers) include politicians, international bankers and mega-corporations with powerful lobbies in government and low visibility power groups behind the scenes;

- In every fight there is a bully who picks the fight and a victim who is forced into the conflict;
- In Iraq, the USA is the bully. In the Holy Land, Israel is the bully and Palestine the victim;
- Two by-products of war are immorality and financial dilution;
- The method of financing wars is always the printing of money, or 'financial dilution';
- It is shortsighted to look for a political solution to serial wars, because political parties are controlled by the same power structure mentioned above;
- Natural disasters are the Warmaker's next best friend and take the place of unnaturally created disasters (wars) as a method of shifting wealth;
- In the USA, the Federal Reserve System is a private (non-government) organization that has been granted an exclusive monopoly to create credit money. The global supply of money is controlled by bankers in London;
- Those with the smallest income and the least capital are the most diluted by this system;
- Every dollar spent in every war must be repaid, because war produces no gain - it only shifts assets. Intelligent investing will not protect you from dilution, because it cannot protect you from the by-product of dilution - war and immorality;
- The war on terrorism is, in fact, a war of dilution. The effects of World War 3 will be felt by the man in the street at an economic level, not a military level;
- Most individuals have not seen these 'self evident truths' simply because the media is controlled by a half dozen Warmaker influenced companies;
- It is unlikely that serial wars, financial dilution, and moral collapse of our age can be avoided because it is the inherent nature of man. There is a deep-rooted need in many powerful leaders to deny the existence of the Positive Universal Force, because if they did not do this, they would have to submit their own behavior-patterns to the instruction set introduced by the Positive Force. This is unacceptable to the Negative Force, hence the giant Cosmic Battle, with ramifications in this dimension.

Because the statements above are self evident truths, there can be no soft landing from the financial and military disaster various parts of the world now face. But financial disaster is less permanent than moral destruction. Our parents survived The Great Depression, and those who are mentally prepared for the next Depression will survive it too.

Let us discuss a few very specific actions one can take if you agree that time is indeed running out.

Self Preservation

The historical average for free societies to move from total freedom to total lockdown is 7 years. The US clock started ticking on September 11, 2001. Using the average of 7 years takes us to September 2008. However, recent developments in the advancement of a police state have moved very quickly, which seems to indicate that Martial Law could be declared in the US sooner than 2008. Martial Law will be introduced in tandem with a collapsing economy and the fictitious Avian Flu.[172] When the US economy falters, the rest of the global economy will follow suit. The writing is on the wall that we are entering a time of great upheaval, perhaps as early as 2006, perhaps as late as 2012.

For the sheeple, life will continue as they have been accustomed to live until they have lost everything. It is difficult to believe, but that is precisely what has happened in every single Depression to date. Known as complacency, this lackadaisical mindset is very often fuelled by an artificially high living standard, thanks to easily available credit prior to the collapse. But when the credit disappears, so will lives.

It is foolish to refuse to prepare for events that are a distinct possibility. It is beyond foolish to see these events approaching and ignore them. As winter arrives, the necessary arrangements are made for warmth. Failure to do so means many months of cold and misery at best, and death by exposure at worst. Failure to prepare for war will mean immense economic hardship at best, and forced labor in concentration camps leading to death at worst.

The question is, What will you do? Having completed this manual the temptation will be strong to slip back into the anti-civilization bubble you have worked so hard to escape from. We hope that is not the path you will choose and encourage you to consider the following actions.

Real Estate

If you currently own real estate in any Western nation, but particularly the US, consider extracting the capital from your property as soon as possible, even if that means selling and renting for the next few years. It is better to sell before the peak than after. We fear the peak has already passed.

---

[172] www.healthliesexposed.com/articles/article_2005_10_14_2714.shtml

"If the American people ever allow private banks to control the issue of their currency, first by inflation, then by deflation, the banks and the corporations which grow up around them will deprive the people of all property until their children wake up homeless on the continent their fathers conquered." – Thomas Jefferson – Founding President of the United States.[173]

Private Banks *do* currently control the issue of currency, through the private Federal Reserve (which is neither Federal, nor a Reserve). Over the past 80 years, inflation and deflation have been introduced in a controlled manner, purely with the intent of 'depriving people of property'.

"A democracy cannot exist as a permanent form of government. It can only exist until the voters discover that they can vote themselves largess from the public treasury. From that time on the majority always votes for the candidates promising the most benefits from the public treasury, with the results that a democracy always collapses over loose fiscal policy, always followed by a dictatorship.

The average age of the world's great civilizations has been 200 years. These nations have progressed through this sequence:
from bondage to spiritual faith
from spiritual faith to great courage
from courage to liberty
from liberty to abundance
from abundance to selfishness
from selfishness to complacency
from complacency to apathy
from apathy to dependency
from dependency back to bondage." - Alexander Fraser Tytler (1742-1813)[174]

It is not difficult to see that many Western nations are at least in the age of apathy, if not total dependency. Look for example at the expectation that governments must assist in any emergency – no longer are individuals willing or able to fend for themselves. The very next stage is bondage.

America is 230 years old in 2006. Where do you think that nation is in that sequence?

Our strong recommendation is to sell any real estate you may have before it is too late.[175]

---

[173] www.ruwart.com/Healing/chap9.html
[174] www.lewrockwell.com/yates/yates91.html. See also *"The Decline and Fall of the Roman Empire"* written in 1788 by Edward Gibbon. The book set forth five basic reasons why great civilizations wither and die. www.ccel.org/g/gibbon/decline

Self Sufficiency

It goes without saying that now is a particularly precarious time to be relying on a salary or on your possibly insufficient retirement plans. Develop the necessary skills to build an alternative income stream as described in this manual. Remember that inaction and procrastination will be your downfall.

Support Groups

Develop a close-knit group of friends who share a similar mindset – a group like this will be invaluable when days become dark. You may wish to join others who have completed this manual in intelligent debate, discussions and questions in our unique Forum.[176]

Get Out Now

In one of the clearest warning signs of what is in store for most Western nations, Dr. Lawrence Britt has examined the fascist regimes of Hitler (Germany), Mussolini (Italy), Franco (Spain), Suharto (Indonesia) and several Latin American regimes. Britt found 14 defining characteristics common to each. The frightening aspect of his study is the presence of these characteristics in most Western 'democracies' today. You can read *The 14 Defining Characteristics Of Fascism*[177] and then decide whether your country is already a fascist state or not.

It appears that the US, UK, Canada, Australia, Israel and many European nations are already fascist. There may be many more.

The dictionary definition of fascism is: 'A system of government marked by centralization of authority under a dictator, stringent socioeconomic controls, suppression of the opposition through terror and censorship, and typically a policy of belligerent nationalism and racism; A political philosophy or movement based on or advocating such a system of government; Oppressive, dictatorial control.'

Simply stated, a fascist government always has one class of citizens that is considered superior to another based upon race, creed, origin or any other arbitrary classification. It is possible to be both a republic and a fascist state. The preferred class lives in a republic while the oppressed class lives in a fascist state.

More than a class system, fascism specifically targets, dehumanizes and aims to destroy those it deems undesirable.

Why all the discussion on fascism?

---

[175] See www.ThreeWorldWars.com/archive/news/real-estate.htm for details.
[176] www.freedomtechnology.org/forum
[177] www.rense.com/general37/fascism.htm

224

Because, whether it is fair or not, we are all deemed undesirable by those who run the world, both seen and unseen. The writing is on the wall for Martial Law to be declared in the US. What will trigger it is any one of a number of scenarios:

- Simultaneous 'terrorist' attacks across the nation;
- Simultaneous 'natural' disasters across the nation;
- The planned outbreak of a deadly virus which will require quarantining of large groups.

Note that these events can be staged, and may occur in unison to enhance the effect of creating fear, panic and pandemonium.

The countries most at risk of implementing Draconian police state laws are the US, the UK and Australia. Europe is not far behind, as is Canada.

If you live in any of these countries, consider relocating to at least 200 miles (300 kilometers) away from any city with a population of more than 1 million. Ideally you should consider leaving your country entirely.

There is no 100% safe and totally immune country to escape to, but some are better than others. Avoid China, Russia, Africa and most South American countries. We recommend SE Asia, specifically:

- Thailand mainland and surrounding islands (Andaman Sea and Gulf of Thailand)
- Malaysia and islands
- Indonesia and islands
- Philippines and islands
- New Zealand and islands
- The islands of Micronesia and Polynesia
- Cambodia and islands
- Laos
- Vietnam and islands
- Myanmar and islands

You will need to do your own research as to which destination suits you better. We can offer some advice and assistance through www.Econocor.com, a company dedicated to providing low-cost affordable housing throughout SE Asia.

Gold

Since 1980, Central Banks in the US and Europe have been selling their gold hordes in order to keep its true value down and therefore an unattractive option for investment. The same method was employed just prior to World War 1 and World War 2. Once economies crash, gold ownership is declared illegal, and the previously sold gold is returned to Central Bankers via wide-scale confiscation.

In the past, wise citizens refused to turn their gold over, even though this act labeled them as criminals. Keep the following Axioms in mind:

Axiom 10 – Morality: Conventional morality is based on arbitrary, man-made, fickle laws.

Axiom 6 – Rules & Regulations: *Fresh Thinkers* live by their own set of rational, coherent and internally generated rules, which may, or may not agree with the externally imposed laws. Sometimes they will, sometimes they will not. They follow these regulations and accept full and total responsibility for their every action.

These wise citizens used their gold, their real money to leave their homelands and relocate to safer countries.

The conversion of your wealth to real money therefore becomes a priority. Remember too that you are converting your assets into wealth so as to be able to escape an economic war and Martial Law. The sooner you act the more real money you will have.

Keep in mind too, that you are not converting your wealth in order to pay your debts, assuming you have chosen to leave your homeland. Even if you have to purchase gold using your instruments of debt (credit cards, mortgage loans, personal loans, etc.) this is what you must do.

In addition, no concern should be given to material possessions, except those that hold the most sentimental value. Your goal is escaping and building a new life all over again somewhere else. Everything of value to your old life should be sold. This will also assist your efforts in being as mobile as possible.

Your one and only objective should be to accumulate as much gold as possible in the shortest amount of time as possible. Once you are safely out of the way of war, then and only then should your thoughts turn back to the accumulation of luxuries.

A reliable gold dealer in the US is International Collectors Associates in Durango CO.[178] Alternatively, do a Google search on "gold bullion dealer" with the name of your city.

Left Behind

Being left behind in a nation under Martial Law should never be your first option – escaping before war arrives on your doorstep should always be your first priority.

But if for whatever reason you did not escape an area which has deteriorated to Martial Law, remember this:

> *"...a human being can alter his life by altering his attitudes of mind."* – William James

---

[178] www.mcalvany.com

Your mental attitude is the most important asset when you find yourself caught up in a war. The essence of your plan should be for survival at any cost and survival entails escape, evasion, concealment and foraging. None of these can be accomplished without planning. In preparing your plan it is best to start with worst case scenarios. What happens if you cannot draw cash because bank accounts have been frozen? What happens if you cannot obtain food because supermarket shelves are empty? What happens if you cannot use your vehicle because gasoline is not available?

You must further be mentally prepared for experiences that, in reality, cannot be prepared for. This may sound like a contradiction, but is rather a statement of fact. How do you prepare to watch as your wife, mother or daughter is raped? How do you prepare to watch the sudden deaths of those closest to you and yet still continue on? How do you walk away from one child lying dead beside the road with no burial or time to mourn while holding the hand of your other child?

While certainly unpleasant, these are the realities of war, and require careful thought and mental discipline and preparation if you are to save yourself and your family.

Please do not take this information as all you will ever need to know. To be fully prepared entails far more detailed research. A good place to start is www.ThreeWorldWars.com/prepare, but even that is only a starting point.

Community Living

The preceding discussion is necessary to explain the state of the world politically, militarily and economically. Much the same as gravity works whether you understand it or not, so the current state of the world is as it is, whether you choose to accept it or not.

While this may be an extremely negative way of viewing current events, the chance to turn hardship into opportunity presents itself in the Freedom Technology Community.

From the days of the hunter-gatherer culture, individual humans have learned that there is strength in numbers and that sharing work and resources can be a good thing. The Latin root munus or gift, brings into the meaning of community the aspect of giving of one's self to others. The balance between self-interest and shared-interests within and among members of a group is the crucial factor in community formation. When enough participants in a group develop an attitude of caring for the well-being of the whole, or the common good, the prospect of community is present.

Whatever drives people to cooperate and collaborate in the first place, is not quite as important in the context of community as what makes them continue to associate. Resilient connections between and among people are what is important in the formation of viable communities. Successful efforts by a mix of participants tend to attract the attention of other less connected individuals who may seek to join the group that is succeeding.

If the sense of community exists, both freedom and security exist as well. The Community then takes on a life of its own, as people become free enough to share and secure enough to get along. This is the spirit of community, and the spirit of the Freedom Technology community. Initially this is a virtual community, meaning we only ever meet online in the Forum.[179] However, as time progresses, intentional communities may develop all over the world.

What is an Intentional Community?

An intentional community[180] is a group of people who have chosen to live with or near enough to each other to carry out their shared lifestyle or common purpose together. Ecovillages are intentional communities that aspire to create a more humane and sustainable way of life. Typically, an ecovillage builds ecologically sustainable housing, grows much of it is own food, recycles waste products harmlessly and generates it is own off-grid power. These are the communities that Freedom Technology encourages. If you have not already done so, we recommend you register[181] your details with Freedom Technology so that we may update you as these plans progress. If you would like to create such a community, please do contact us so that discussions may commence.

Wrapping Up

We have reached the end of our journey together, but the start of a whole new life, filled with purpose. As you contemplate what the future holds for you, remember this little saying:

> *"Life is not a journey to the grave with the intent of arriving in a pretty and well-preserved body, but rather to skid in broadside, thoroughly used up, worn out, and loudly proclaim 'Wow, what a ride!'"* – Author Unknown

---

[179] www.freedomtechnology.org/forum
[180] http://en.wikipedia.org/wiki/Intentional_Community
[181] www.freedomtechnology.org/forum

21. Appendix A – Finding the Old & Young Woman

This explanation is to assist in finding either the old or young woman. Read the relevant description below and then go back to page 16 to see if you can find her.

Old Woman: She is looking slightly down towards your left, with her chin tucked into her neck. The young woman's choker is her mouth. The young woman's cheek-line and chin is her nose. The young woman's ear is her eye.

Young Woman: She is looking away from you towards your left. The old woman's mouth is a choker around her slender neck. The old woman's nose is her cheek-line and chin (looking away from you). The old woman's left eye is her left ear.

22. Appendix B – Suggested Wedding Vows

[Man] and [Woman] have not come here today to make a solemn promise or to exchange a sacred vow.

[Woman] and [Man] have come here to make public their love for each other; to declare their choice to live and partner and grow together – out loud and in your presence, out of their desire that we will all come to feel a very real and intimate part of their decision, and thus make it even more powerful.

They have also come here today in the further hope that their ritual of bonding will help bring us all closer together. If you are here today with a spouse or partner, let this ceremony be a reminder – a rededication of your own loving bond.

We will begin by asking the question: Why get married? [Man] and [Woman] have answered this question for themselves. Now I want to ask them one more time, so they can be sure of their answer, certain of their understanding, and firm in their commitment to the truth they share.

(Person leading the ceremony lifts two Red Roses)

This is the Ceremony of Roses, in which [Woman] and [Man] share their understandings, and commemorate that sharing.

Now [Man] and [Woman], you have told me it is your firm understanding that you are not entering into this marriage for reasons of security.

That the only real security is not in owning or possessing, nor being owned or possessed.

Not in demanding or expecting, and not even in hoping, that what you think you need in life will be supplied by the other; but rather, in knowing that everything you need in life - all the love, all the wisdom, all the insight, all the power, all the knowledge, all the understanding, all the nurturing, all the compassion, and all the strength - resides within you; and that you are not each marrying the other in hopes of getting these things, but in hopes of giving these gifts, that the other might have them in even greater abundance.

Is that your firm understanding today?

(Appropriate response from couple e.g. "It is".)

[Woman] and [Man], you have told me it is your firm understanding you are not entering into this marriage as a means of in any way limiting, controlling, hindering or restricting each other from any true expression and honest celebration of that which is the highest and best within you – including your love of God, your love of life, your love of people, your love of creativity, your love of work, or any aspect of your being which genuinely represents you, and brings you joy.

Is that still your firm understanding today?

(Appropriate response from couple e.g. "It is".)

Further [Man] and [Woman], you have told me it is your firm understanding that you are not entering into this marriage in the blind belief that it will miraculously last forever, based purely on the traditions of a promise. You acknowledge that a fulfilled relationship requires both partners to agree that the mutual and honest exchange of each other's contribution to the relationship will lead to a temporary increase in happiness for both partners.

If any promise is to be made today, it is that you both promise to acknowledge the ongoing need for mutual and honest exchanges of value in the relationship. You both absolve each other of any ongoing commitment if the current approximately equal exchange of values becomes imbalanced.

Is that still your firm understanding today?

(Appropriate response from couple e.g. "It is".)

Finally, [Man] and [Woman], you have said to me that you do not see marriage as producing obligations, but rather as providing opportunities - opportunities for growth, for full self-expression, for lifting your lives to their highest potential, for healing every false thought or small idea you ever had about yourself, and for the communion of your two souls.

You are starting a journey through life with one you love as an equal partner, sharing equally both the authority and the responsibilities inherent in any partnership, bearing equally what burdens there be, basking equally in the glories.

Is that the vision you wish to enter into now?

(Appropriate response from couple e.g. "It is".)

I now give you these Red Roses, symbolizing your individual understandings of these Earthly things; that you both know and agree how life will be with you in bodily form, and within the physical structure called marriage. Give these Roses now to each other as a symbol of your sharing of these agreements and understandings with love.

(Person leading the ceremony lifts two White Roses, up side down, with a ring on each stem).

Now, please each of you take this White Rose. It is a symbol of your larger understandings, of your spiritual nature and your spiritual truth. It stands for the purity of your Real and Highest Self, and of the purity of God's love, which shines upon you now and always.

(Rose with appropriate ring given to [Man] and [Woman]).

Suggested Wedding Vows

What symbols do you bring as a reminder of the promises given and received today?

([Man] and [Woman] remove the rings from the rose stems and give them to person leading the ceremony, who holds them in hand and says...)

A circle is the symbol of the Sun, and the Earth, and the Universe. It is a symbol of holiness, and of perfection and peace. It is also the symbol of eternality of spiritual truth, love, and life...
That which has no beginning and no end. And in this moment, [Woman] and [Man] choose for it to also be a symbol of unity, but not of possession, of joining, but not of restricting, of encirclement, but not of entrapment. For love cannot be possessed, nor can it be restricted. And the soul can never be entrapped. Now [Man] and [Woman], please take these rings you wish to give, one to the other.

([Man] and [Woman] take each other's rings).

[Man], please repeat after me.

I, [Man]...ask you, [Woman] to be my partner, my lover, my friend and my wife...I announce and declare my intention to give you my deepest friendship and love...not only when your moments are high...but when they are low...not only when you remember clearly Who You Are...but when you forget...not only when you are acting with love...but when you are not...I further announce...before God and those here present...that I will seek always to see the Light of Divinity within you...and seek always to share...the Light of Divinity within me...even, and especially...in whatever moments of darkness may come.

It is my intention to be with you forever...in a Partnership of the Soul...that we may do together God's work...sharing all that is good within us...with all those whose lives we touch.

[Woman], do you wish to grant [Man]'s request that you be his wife?

(I do)

Now [Woman], please repeat after me.

I, [Woman]...ask you, [Man] to be my partner, my lover, my friend and my husband...I announce and declare my intention to give you my deepest friendship and love...not only when your moments are high...but when they are low...not only when you remember clearly Who You Are...but when you forget...not only when you are acting with love...but when you are not...I further announce...before God and those here present...that I will seek always to see the Light of Divinity within you...and seek always to share...the Light of Divinity within me...even, and especially...in whatever moments of darkness may come.

232

It is my intention to be with you forever...in a Partnership of the Soul...that we may do together God's work...sharing all that is good within us...with all those whose lives we touch.

[Man], do you choose to grant [Woman]'s request that you be her husband?

(I do)

Please then, both of you take the rings you would give each other, and repeat after me:

With this ring I thee wed...I take now the ring you give to me...and give it place upon my hand...that all may see and know...of my love for you.

We recognize with full awareness that only a couple can administer the sacrament of marriage to each other, and only a couple can sanctify it. Neither myself, nor any power invested in me by the State, can grant me the authority to declare what only two hearts can declare, and what only two souls can make real. And so now, inasmuch as you, [Woman], and you [Man], have announced the truths that are already written in your hearts, and have witnessed the same in the presence of these, your friends and children, and of the One True God – we observe joyfully that you have declared yourself to be Husband and Wife.

Let us now join in prayer.

Spirit of Love and Life: out of this whole world, two souls have found each other.

Their destinies shall now be woven into one design, and their perils and their joys shall not be known apart. [Man] and [Woman], may your home be a place of happiness for all who enter it; a place where the old and the young are renewed in each other's company, a place for growing and a place for sharing, a place for music and a place for laughter, a place for prayer and a place for love. May the beauty and the bounty of your love for one another constantly enrich those who are nearest to you, may your work be a joy of your life that serves the world, and may your days be good and long upon the Earth.
Amen.

23. Appendix C – The Fresh Wisdom Axioms

Axiom #1 – Reducing Controls

In order to become free, *Fresh Thinkers* greatly reduce the external controls placed on their life. They will not allow themselves to be controlled by anyone (including Freedom Technology and the authors of *Fresh Wisdom*). They recognize the various controlling tactics for what they are, and will not allow them to influence their life negatively.

Axiom #2 – Avoid Con Artists

Con artists seek to maximize the volume of life's pleasures which flow their way, by conning money, energy, time and talent from other people. By bending the talents, energy and time of the mass of people to their will, such individuals and organizations seek to profit with minimum effort on their part. *Fresh Thinkers* understand this and avoid Con Artists.

Axiom #3 – Recognizing Illusions

Fresh Thinkers make it a lifelong task to continually unmask the illusions created by others. The extent to which they believe in one or more of the illusions is the extent to which they are still enslaved. The facets of life which are home to the greatest number of illusions are:
1. Health and Longevity
2. Relationships and Romantic Love
3. Religion
4. Finance, Money and Wealth Creation
5. Personal Freedom

There are, of course, many other minor illusions, but your knowledge of the five main categories of illusions will provide you with the information required to tackle the smaller and less significant ones. Remember – the illusions are the vehicles which people who want something from you use to extract your time, money and talents.

Axiom #4 – All Are Not Equal

Very few people will choose the path of freedom and unlimited personal power in their lives. In this respect, all are created equal in the options available to them, but not all make the same (equal) choices in life.

As *Fresh Thinkers*, we recognize this inequality, and will not attempt to convince the sheep of the value of this lifestyle. We realize this is an impossible and thankless task.

Axiom #5 – Altruism

True altruism does exist, but is so rare that it can be ignored for all intents and purposes. By true altruism, we mean an act which is entirely selfless with absolutely no pay-off of any description.

Axiom #6 – Rules and Regulations

Fresh Thinkers live by their own set of rational, coherent and internally generated rules, which may, or may not agree with the externally imposed laws. Sometimes they will, sometimes they will not. They follow these regulations and accept full and total responsibility for their every action. They also accept the consequences on a strict cause and effect basis, if these actions happen to conflict with the law of the land at a particular time, and in a particular place. We have no opinion on the fairness of any particular law, since we know that all laws are more or less arbitrary and 'unfair'.

Axiom #7 – Fairness

The world is, and always has been, an unfair place. *Fresh Thinkers* know this, and do not find it surprising. They do not squander their life-energies in an attempt to change this situation.

The statement "It is not fair!" comes only from the mouth of a sheep that is controlled by the law, and is whining because the rules are not tight enough. Someone has slipped through the net, and the sheep want the net closed.

Axiom #8 – Purpose

The uninitiated masses almost never know their real reasons for doing anything. *Fresh Thinkers*, in contrast, never accept anything without questioning and understanding it. They also understand that their life has a purpose, even though their purpose may not yet have been fully defined or understood.

Axiom #9 – Religion

Religions and cults are man-made inventions designed to allow an elitist priesthood to con value out of those that follow them. *Fresh Thinkers* do not blindly follow any man-made religion.

Axiom #10 – Morality

Conventional morals are purely influenced by the latitude and longitude at which you happen to find yourself, together with the date currently showing on your calendar. In other words, laws are applicable to the country you happen to be in at a specific time. It is likely that those laws were different in the past and do not currently apply to other locations. This means that conventional morality is based on arbitrary, man-made, fickle laws. The morals of a *Fresh Thinker* are not based on man-made laws but are instead internally generated, according to the Immutable Laws of Nature.

Axiom #11 – Responsibility

Responsibility for what happens in the life of a *Fresh Thinker* rests solely with that person. This is particularly true when known laws are transgressed, and we do not question the fairness or otherwise of the consequences.

Axiom #12 – Relationships

Successful relationships hinge upon a continued and approximately equal exchange of values between the partners. When an imbalance occurs a *Fresh Thinker* either addresses the imbalance or ends the relationship.

Axiom # 13 – Biblical World View

A *Fresh Thinker* accepts without question the Biblical World View and that the only scientifically, empirically proven source document is the Bible. This book is not at variance with any proven scientific fact and shows an internal concordance of knowledge of the world of science which the initial writers could not have had, except for its inspiration by an Outside Mind. The Biblical World View is thus the only scientifically proven paradigm (way of looking at life), and thus represents a stable pyramid.

Axiom # 14 – Modern Science Distorts the Biblical Message

A *Fresh Thinker* understands that the theme of the Bible is that of a gigantic Cosmic conflict between positive and negative forces. We therefore accept that any distortion of the Biblical World View is accomplished by negative forces intent on preventing the achievement of a personal Omega Point.

24. Appendix D – Further Reading

The following websites are recommended to the reader for additional background and specific information on the various topics covered in this book.

Since changes on the web occur frequently, some links may be out of date. All links are maintained and may be accessed at **www.FreedomTechnology.org/links**.

Because content on the web can frequently change, the authors do not vouch for the ongoing integrity of each link mentioned. The reader is encouraged to question everything online, and to listen for the ring of truth.

The Power of a Paradigm page 16

www.taketheleap.com/define.html - A simple definition for a Paradigm Shift.

www.michaelbrown.org/html/transformations.html - A more detailed explanation of Paradigm Shifts. This article examines processes that expand and transform consciousness.

www.unveilingthem.com/SecretCovenant.htm – The secret covenant against all humanity. Reading this disturbing document will give you a clearer understanding of why the world is in the state it is.

www.secretsocieties.net/whoswho.htm– Who's Who of the Elite by Robert Gaylon Ross, Sr. The worldwide Elite oligarchy has decided that the public is "on-to-them" when they use the term "New World Order", so they have changed the code words to "GLOBAL". When you hear them use such terms as Global architecture, Global economy, Global village, Global interests, Global neighborhood, Global movement, Global needs, and the like, you can substitute the old code name of New World Order, and you will know that they are still talking about the secret cabal that is trying to dominate economic and political control of the ENTIRE world.

www.thewatcherfiles.com/bloodlines/ - The 13 Satanic Bloodlines. The light of truth in this book will be too bright for some people who will want to return to the safe comfort of their darkness. I am not a conspiracy theorist. I deal with real facts, not theory. Some of the people I write about, I have met. Some of the people I expose are alive and very dangerous. The darkness has never liked the light.

www.mega.nu:8080/ampp/ - The Architecture of Modern Political Power - An understanding of cultural context is prerequisite to meaningful discussion and contemplation of the architecture of modern political power. Out of this context comes the vocabulary of subjection. The long and sordid history of autocracy is clear enough — such regimes are little more than naïve scale-ups of tribal society, intellectually easy to dismiss, and with the proliferation of alternative systems, easy to oust because unpopular.

~~~

The Immutable Laws of Nature page 21

www.yesselman.com – A dedication to Baruch Spinoza with his Universal Man.

http://plato.stanford.edu/entries/kant-moral - Kant's Moral Philosophy. Kant argued that moral requirements are based on a standard of rationality he dubbed the "Categorical Imperative" (CI). Immorality thus involves a violation of the CI and is thereby irrational.

~~~

How Media Molds Our Minds page 30

www.cjr.org/tools/owners - Columbia Journalism Review's online guide to what major media companies own. Includes a selected list of articles about media ownership.

www.lewrockwell.com/orig2/liebermann1.html – How Propaganda Works in the 21st Century

www.freedomtechnology.org/resources/altmedia.htm - Reliable alternative media sources.

~~~

Ultimate Health & Longevity page 44 and 136

www.healingdaily.com/beliefs.htm - Further examples of how the medical industry influences public opinion.

www.healthliesexposed.com/articles/article_2005_08_19_3132.shtml - 8 Medical Lies and Why I Abandoned Medicine by Shane Ellison, dedicated to stopping the prescription drug hype in its tracks.

www.drcranton.com/chelation.htm - A good source of information to start researching Chelation Therapy.

www.lef.org - The Life Extension Foundation

www.maxlife.org - Maximum Life Foundation. Accelerating progress in Anti-Aging Medicine Research

www.acam.org - The American College for Advancement in Medicine (ACAM) is a not-for-profit medical society dedicated to educating physicians and other health care professionals on the latest findings and emerging procedures in preventive/nutritional medicine. ACAM's goals are to improve skills, knowledge and diagnostic procedures as they relate to complementary and alternative medicine; to support research; and to develop awareness of alternative methods of medical treatment.

www.archive.org/details-db.php?mediatype=movies&identifier=ChelationTherapyRevolutio n - 'Chelation Therapy Revolution' (describes use of EDTA as a chelating agent, 1999)

www.cleanse.net/mucoid_plaque.HTM – Articles by Dr. Richard Anderson, author of Cleanse and Purify Thyself Volume 1 & 2.

http://educate-yourself.org/nwo/nwopopcontrol.shtml – Article explaining the plan to intentionally reduce the bulk of the world's population through genocide via the introduction of population slaughter, orchestrated conflicts, and bioengineered disease organisms introduced via vaccines and other means of external transmission.

http://fatima.freehosting.net/Articles/Art3.htm – A collection of quotes from Advocates of Population Reduction.

www.generationrescue.org – Parent-led advocacy group promoting use of chelation therapy as a cure for autism.

www.healingcelebrations.com/SARS.htm – SARS: The Great Global Scam.

www.marthavolchok.com - Colon Cleanse for Radiant Health

www.blessedherbs.com/photos2i.html - Real pictures of colon plaque eliminated during a Colon Cleansing Therapy Session (not for the faint-hearted!)

www.mcguffmedical.com - All requirements for doing EDTA Chelation can be obtained directly from McGuff Medical Products.

www.originofaids.com – Provides scientific background on the link between the hepatitis B vaccine and the AIDS pandemic.

www.sciencedaily.com/upi/index.php?feed=Science&article=UPI-1-20050524-16281400-bc-ageofautism-chelation.xml - 'The Age of Autism: Heavy Metal', Dan Olmsted (May 24, 2005)
www.snopes.com/toxins/fecal.htm – The other side of the coin: a large number of articles covering the misunderstood negative side of colon cleansing.

http://sites.securemc.com/folder21885/index.cfm?id=50&fuseaction=browse&pageid=40 – This article on the True Nature of Cancer is required reading for anyone facing cancer.

www.wealth4freedom.com/truth/7/uselesseaters.htm – Article on eliminating the useless eaters through population control.

www.worldpsychology.net/World Psychology/SaudeVeritas/IDCC.htm - International Detoxification and Chelation Clinic

www.gen.cam.ac.uk/sens/ - Expediting the development of a true cure for human aging.

www.alcor.org – Alcor Life Extension Foundation.

~~~

Independent Wealth Creation page 57, 149 and 216
http://web.archive.org/web/20040226162618/www.wealthstudy.com/studentsonly/Strategic_Wealth/toc.htm - Strategic Wealth Home Study Course

www.buildfreedom.com/tl/rape1.shtml – The Economic Rape of America

www.lewrockwell.com/yates/yates91.html - The Coming Financial Train Wreck - Large parts of economics are not hard to figure out – to a logical mind, that is. This is because economics is a real world application of a more basic and very powerful subject: deductive logic.

www.conspiracypenpal.com/columns/gold.htm - What is Gold Really Worth Today? - "By this means (fractional reserve banking) government may secretly and unobserved, confiscate the wealth of the people, and not one man in a million will detect the theft." ---The Economic Consequences of the Peace, John Maynard Keynes (the father of Keynesian Economics) (1920)

www.MillionDollarDay.com – John Reese, and Internet entrepreneur, who was the first to make sales of more than $1m in 24 hours in mid-2004.

http://web.archive.org/web/20041011160453/http://www.solgroup.com/notax/index.html - How to stop paying Federal Income Tax – legally.

~~~

Spiritual and Metaphysical Truths page 69, 107 and 164

www.infidels.org/library/modern/james_haught/holy.html – A record of bloody battles fought through the ages, triggered by, or attributable to various religions.

http://johnnyskeptic.com/ – The author raises a number of valid concerns, while calling into question a number of fundamentalist Christian claims. However, this is a perfect example of someone who hasn't understood the true meaning of the Bible and instead spends their time debating often meaningless 'issues'.

www.experiencefestival.com/a/ChristianFaith/id/50216 – How does one define reality from the perspective of faith? St Anselm defines theology as "faith seeking understanding". St Augustine, citing Plato, argued for the necessity of eternal, universal spiritual principles and laws on which our contingent and temporal realm of existence is based. For Augustine, God is the author and overseer of these principles and laws.

http://web.archive.org/web/20041020015016/www.counterpunch.org/mcguire0810.html – A skeptic's view of Christianity. "If you probe many sincere Christians you often discover oily wells of anger, inferiority, guilt and shame. The religion seems to create and nourish underground oceans of the stuff. I started calling Christianity the Snake With the Magic Tail. The snake has its fangs buried in your neck (the shame and guilt) but if you bite down hard enough on the snake's magic tail (absolute faith) it withdraws the fangs a little, and your pain is relieved (forgiveness). It is a whole system, but Christians do not see the connections."

www.abarim-publications.com/artbintro.html – An Introduction to Biblical Scripture Theory. Scripture Theory is to texts what Chaos Theory is to creation. Scripture Theory tries to isolate patterns in the narrative, in order to understand it better and to finally arrive at some kind of system that describes the principles of a text's governing dynamics. The difference between a book and a great book is often the consistency of patterns in the latter.

www.bible.org/page.asp?page_id=42 – The Creation of the Heavens and the Earth, using Chaos Theory.

www.chemistry.ohio-state.edu/betha/qm/ - An introduction to the principles of Quantum Mechanics.

http://higgo.com/quantum/laymans.htm – A Lazy Layman's Guide to Quantum Physics.

www.meta-library.net/physics/qmprovid-body.html – God's Providence and Quantum Mechanics

www.reasons.org/resources/apologetics/quantummech.shtml – Quantum Mechanics and the Bible. The Bible speaks of the existence of dimensions beyond our time and space, extra dimensions in which God exists and operates. Such extra dimensions are now verified by scientific discoveries.

www.spaceandmotion.com/ - The Dynamic Unity of Reality. An excellent website, albeit a little disorganized, explaining Truth and Reality from a Scientific perspective.

www.physics-philosophy-metaphysics.com/forum/ - Physics, Philosophy and Metaphysics Forum – The discussions here will blow your mind! The purpose of this Forum is to discuss the Wave Structure of Matter (WSM) which is summarized in the main Forum sections on Index page. This work is still in the early stages of development, both in terms of knowledge, and in getting this knowledge out into the world. Significantly, by describing Reality most simply, in terms of One thing existing, Space, with Properties of a Continuous Infinite Eternal Wave Medium, the Wave Structure of Matter (WSM) explains and solves many of the fundamental problems of Science (Metaphysics

Philosophy Physics) by explaining how matter (and thus humans) are necessarily interconnected to other matter in Space within the Universe. We think this knowledge is important, hope that you find it interesting and will enjoy pondering upon this new perspective for understanding physical reality.

www.everystudent.com/features/connecting.html – Connecting With the Divine. A look into the major world faith systems: Hinduism, New Age, Buddhism, Islam, and Christianity. Included is a brief description of each, its distinguishing characteristics, and what a person can gain from each. The author then presents for your consideration the ways in which Jesus' teaching differs from the world's religions.

www.allaboutthejourney.org/evidence-for-intelligent-design.htm – Evidence for Intelligent Design. Sir Arthur Keith, a famous British evolutionary anthropologist and anatomist, declares: "Evolution is unproved and unprovable. We believe it only because the only alternative is special creation, and that is unthinkable."

www.allaboutgod.com/does-god-exist.htm – Does God Exist Scientifically? There are many scientific discoveries you will not learn about from high school and college textbooks. The best-known "icons" of evolution – from pictures of apes evolving into humans, to comparisons of fish and human embryos, to moths on tree trunks – are fraudulent or misleading. For decades, biology students have been taught things about evolution that are simply untrue. Wait until you start reading some of the truth… it is utterly amazing…

www.godandscience.org/cults/index.html – Aberrant "Christian" Theology.

www.godandscience.org/apologetics/bibletru.html – Is the Bible Really the Word of God? John Warwick Montgomery tells us a parable: "A great king (God) had a son (mankind) who had grown up out of contact with his father. While journeying in a distant province the son fell seriously ill. The doctor accompanying him (reason) was incapable of treating the disease, but the king, learning of his son's plight, sent instructions (the gospel) for the healing of the boy. However, the king's numerous enemies also discovered what had happened, and they likewise sent remedies – purporting to come from the king – which were actually poisonous (non-Christian religious and philosophical options). The son's solution to this dilemma was to evaluate the remedies by three tests: first, what each remedy revealed about his father (comparison being made with the likeness to the father possessed by the son himself); second, how accurately each remedy pictured the nature of the disease; and thirdly, how sound the various curative methods appeared to be. With the help of the doctor, the son finally made his decision in terms of the remedy that best satisfied all three tests."

www.clarifyingchristianity.com/science.shtml – Science and the Bible. The Bible is not a science book, yet it is scientifically accurate. We are not aware of any scientific evidence that contradicts the Bible. We have listed statements on this page that are consistent with known scientific facts. Many of them were listed in the Bible hundreds or even thousands of years before being recorded elsewhere.

www.newspeakdictionary.com/ct-matrix.html – A few random observations on The Quantum and Political Mechanics of the movie, The Matrix.

http://answers.google.com/answers/threadview?id=272824 – What is The Matrix? Interesting links provided by one of the Google researchers.

http://web.archive.org/web/20041127093007/http:/www.math.tulane.edu/~tipler/summary.html – Frank J. Tippler's Essays – on The Omega Point.

www.truebiblecode.com – An alternative view to Michael Drosnin's *The Bible Code.*

www.bibleandscience.com - The Institute for Biblical and Scientific Studies is a non-profit tax-exempt organization interested in the areas of Bible and science. The goals of the Institute are to educate people about Bible and science and to do research in Bible and science.

www.blavatsky.net/blavatsky/arts/WhatIsTruth.htm - What is Truth?

www.lifeandtruth.com/truth.htm - The truth about absolute truth.

http://forums.philosophyforums.com/thread/9096 - Debate: Whether there exists absolute truth

www.poyl.com – How to Find the Purpose of Your Life

~~~

Fascinating Relationships page 38 and 115

www.fascinatingwomanhood.net – Marriage, the Fascinating Way, by Helen Andelin. "I know that men are also at fault for marriage problems, but I also know that women working alone can bring about dramatic changes in marriage by following laws of the Universe discovered and taught by Sir Isaac Newton."

www.savethemales.ca/001170.html - The Hoax of Female Empowerment – A powerful article explaining the bigger picture of the destruction of the family unit. "The purpose of female empowerment is to dissolve the family and to increase our dependence on the media and government, which are both owned and controlled by agents of Illuminist bankers." Be sure to read all the comments sent in by readers, male and female.

~~~

Personal Freedom and Sovereignty page 86

www.wealth4freedom.com/truth/links2educate.htm - An extensive list of freedom related reading material to educate yourself on your rights as a Sovereign Individual.

www.lawfulpath.com - Dedicated to study of the True Law, and a return to Lawful Government.

www.worldnewsstand.net/guns/truth.htm - A table explaining the difference between the Republic of the United States and the modern day Corporation it has become and what this means to your personal sovereignty.

~~~

The Freedom Technology Community page 220

www.econocor.com – Established by the founders of Freedom Technology, Econocor builds (to specification) low-cost alternative accommodation throughout South East Asia.

www.ecobooks.com/catalogs/cohousing.htm - Books on Community Living

www.holocaustsurvivors.org/survivors.shtml – Excellent lessons in survival from those who survived concentration camps in the early 1940's.

25. Appendix E – Freedom Technology Web Pages

What is Freedom Technology all about?
www.FreedomTechnology.org/overview.htm

Where can I find out about more Freedom Technology and the people behind the company?
www.FreedomTechnology.org/about.htm

I have further questions – where can I go for answers?
www.FreedomTechnology.org/faq.htm

Where can I interact with other *Fresh Thinkers*?
www.FreedomTechnology.org/forum

How do I contact Freedom Technology?
www.FreedomTechnology.org/contact

I'd like to tell my friends and family about Fresh Wisdom – how do I do that?
www.FreedomTechnology.org/tellfriends

I'm interested in taking the Fresh Wisdom principles further – can you recommend other resources?
www.freedomtechnology.org/resources

Where can I find out more about a long-term plan to change society's perceptions?
www.ThreeWorldWars.com

3126